Medical Investigations

A Book to Inspire Your Interest in Medicine & How Doctors Think

By Dr. Russ Hill & Dr. Richard Griffith

Medical Investigation 101

Copyright ©2017 Hill & Griffith

All Rights Reserved

No part of this book may be reproduced in any form or by any electronic or mechanical means, including information storage and retrieval systems, without permission in writing from the publisher, except by reviewers, who may quote brief passages in a review.

Written and Published by

Dr. Russ Hill

Laguna Beach, CA

and

Dr. Richard Griffith

Guilford, Vermont

Artwork images by Raella Hill

Laguna Beach, CA

Acknowledgements

My occupation as an educator, teaching a newly developed class in pre-medical science, provided the motivation to create a textbook specifically for my students. I also hope this material can encourage other young people to consider a career in healthcare. If the book does not prove that successful, I still expect each reader to make better choices when they themselves need medical attention. Without the collaboration of my cousin and co-author, Dr. Richard Griffith, this endeavor would not have been completed. His medical practice experiences proved indispensable.

We are indebted to language arts teacher Veronica LaFrossia for reading our early material and guiding us to a more interesting and informative presentation style for the students for whom we wrote this book.

We also owe thanks to our early student readers, Pauline Le, Ashley Hernandez, and Nina Le, who encouraged us eagerly to turn out another chapter quickly for them to devour. We thank 6th grade student Grettee Pham for her creatively designed "Lifestyle Suggestions" flow map in chapter 3.6B. We also owe thanks to my 2016-2017 STEM students, who utilized the book and assignments in class, pointing out typographical errors and omissions along the way. That proved they actually read every page and they clearly made this a much better book.

Finally, thanks must go to the writers' spouses, Raella and Claire, for putting up with our time away from family, trading copious emails back and forth across the country. Special thanks to my wife, Raella, not only for reading and editing our material, but especially for the incredible artwork that makes key material visual.

And, of course, thank you, our newest reader, for your interest in learning about how physicians approach medical investigations. We hope we have provided you an unexpected adventure.

Dr. Russ Hill

Medical Investigation 101

Dear Reader:

As you read through the book you will notice highlighted key words. The key words provide opportunities to build your medical vocabulary. We encourage you to learn and remember as much medical terminology as possible, not only for your future career in healthcare, but so you better understand things you hear when you visit your doctor now. Having the ability to communicate effectively with your physician can assist him or her to better diagnose your medical problems and provide you optimum health.

We encourage you to keep a pencil or pen handy when reading our book. You will encounter questions throughout your reading that ask you to think about or write down your thoughts. Should you desire a more interactive experience, we invite you to purchase the *Medical Investigation 101 Workbook*. The workbook challenges your understanding of the medical vocabulary and pulls together the principles presented in your reading. On completion of the workbook you are entitled to hang on your wall an impressive, fun Certificate of Achievement clipped from the back of the workbook that will impress your friends and make your parents very proud. For teachers, *Medical Investigation 101 Teacher's Edition* provides the preferred answers to the questions, crossword puzzles, and activities presented in the workbook.

Table of Contents

Introduction 1
Investigation 1.1: Types of Medical Doctors 5
Investigation 1.2: The Medical Support Team 13
Investigation 1.2B: Medical Support Team Referrals 16
Investigation 2: Medical Diagnostic Process 19
2.0: Introduction: The Medical Diagnostic Process 20
Investigation 2.1: Chief Complaint 23
Investigation 2.2: The Medical History 25
Investigation 2.3: Review of Systems 29
Investigation 2.4: Medical Examination 31
Investigation 2.5: Differential Diagnosis 34
Investigation 2.6: The Diagnosis 36
Investigation 2.7: Soap Notes 40
Investigation 3.1A: Breathing Difficulty 46
Investigation 3.1B: Pulmonary Embolism 48
Investigation 3.2A: Abdominal Pain 51
Investigation 3.2B: Microbes 62-
Investigation 3.3A: Rib Area Pain 74
Investigation 3.4A: Sore Throat 83
Investigation 3.4B: The Role of Blood 89
Investigation 3.5A: Emergencies 97
Investigation 3.5B: Chest Pain 102
Investigation 3.6A: Chronic Disease 106
Investigation 3.6B: Diabetes 113
Investigation 3.7A: Shoulder Pain 122
Investigation 3.7B: Joints 129

Investigation 3.8A: Fever and Cough 134
Investigation 3.8B: Respiratory System 144
Investigation 3.9A: Abdominal Pain and Dark Urine 150
Investigation 3.9B: Urinary Tract 158
Investigation 3.10A: Weak and Dizzy 164
Investigation 3.10B: Environmental Toxins 173
Investigation 3.11A: Food-borne Illness 179
Investigation 3.11B: Foodborne Pathogen Case 189
Investigation 3.12A: Head Injury 192
Investigation 3.12B: The Eye 200
Investigation 3.13A: The Brain 210
Investigation 3.13B: Normal or Abnormal? 220
Investigation 3.14A: Final Case 230
Investigation 3.14B: Circle of Life 235
Investigation 3.15: Looking Deeper 238
Post-Script 244
About the Authors: 245

Introduction

On becoming a medical detective...

Welcome to the challenging world of **medical investigation**. This world has many players but **medical doctors**, also known as **physicians** or **practitioners**, use medical science to care for patients. As you will soon see, there are many ways doctors help people by using their knowledge of the human body and disease. Think about your last visit to your doctor. Physicians who care for children we call **Pediatricians**. **Family physicians** treat family members of all ages, and other doctors called **specialists** treat more complex medical problems, but within a much more limited spectrum of illness or body system. Some doctors work behind the scenes to help patients whom they never meet. You will learn about some of them later.

Medical detectives use a process very similar to crime scene investigators or any other investigator. Solving a medical puzzle requires finding the cause of the problem, the **diagnosis**, and a solution to make the patient feel better, the **treatment.** In spite of learning all they can from the patient and looking at test results, sometimes doctors have a tough time making the **diagnosis**.

The practice of medicine is very much an **art** as much as it is a **science**. The art of medical practice requires scientific knowledge of chemistry, physics, physiology, pathophysiology, and anatomy, but also a sense within the practitioner of human nature and a will to deal with his or her fellow humans in a caring and forgiving manner.

We call the details about how the human body normally works **physiology**. We call the details of how that process can go wrong **pathophysiology**; the Greek word "**path**" means a feeling or an illness. We call a physician who looks for abnormal human **tissue** under a microscope or with chemical tests in the laboratory a **Pathologist**. All **medical investigators** must understand physiology and pathophysiology to do the detective work required to help their patients. We want to introduce you to the art and science, and adventure, of being a **medical detective**.

Detectives start with a mystery and gather clues to figure out what happened and who caused the trouble. Like a detective solving a mystery, doctors start with what they know, add information by **examining** the patient, perhaps giving the patient some tests to get even more information. When they have all the information they can gather, only then can they solve the puzzle and make a diagnosis. For a medical detective the mystery usually starts with a complaint of pain or a change in how the patient feels. Sometimes patients are unable to tell their doctor about their complaint because they are not conscious. When this happens, doctors may have to rely only on their examination of the patient.

Medical Investigation 101

The first clues for solving a medical investigation usually come when the patient tells the story of their complaint or illness. We call the patient's story the **history**. Listening to the history the doctor learns how their health status has changed. We call these changes **symptoms**. Symptoms are not the cause of the problem, but signs that something **abnormal** may be going on. Symptoms give the doctor an idea of where to focus attention.

The physical examination follows, with special attention to areas of pain, discoloration, or swelling related to the complaint. Additional clues come from **X-rays** or **laboratory tests**, such as looking at blood cells under a microscope. We call these additional ways to gather clues **diagnostic testing**. For example, if a patient complains to the doctor of pain in their arm following a fall, an x-ray may show the presence or absence of a break in the bone, called a **fracture**, which cannot be seen using only our eyes.

Physicians and nurse practitioners go through years of training to learn how to **diagnose** the causes of health problems and to become experienced in solving those problems. In this book we hope to provide you a taste of the process and allow you to experience the challenge of using your skills of **observation** and **analysis** to solve the same puzzles that allow doctors and nurses to improve the quality of people's lives. If you feel some frustration in trying to understand everything you need to know to solve these problems, you will not be alone. The best medical specialists in the world share that same frustration, and they **acknowledge** that frustration keeps them studying and learning every day.

Understanding medical investigation is like any new interest; you need to know what things are called and how they work. Medicine has literally thousands of unique terms and probably almost as many processes. This book will introduce many names and many medical procedures, so you may often need to go to books or the Internet to fully satisfy your curiosity. When you dive deeper into understanding medical investigation the learning process really becomes fun and what you learn will stick with you. You are ready to become a Medical Detective. So let's get started!

Investigation 1:
The Medical Team

1.1: Types of Medical Doctors
1.2: Medical Support Team

Investigation 1.1: Types of Medical Doctors

Have you watched an old cowboy movie? Back in the time of the "wild west" anyone shot in a gunfight or banged up in a fistfight got dragged off to the "Doc." The town seemed to have only one "Doc." If a gambler or gunslinger got shot during the time the "Doc" was delivering a baby out at the Ferguson spread, for example, the fate of that gunslinger often proved sub-optimal, if you know what I mean.

Today, if you or I fall sick or are injured we have a variety of types of doctors we might elect to have patch us up. Why do we need so many? What was wrong with the old system where a single doctor took care of whatever folks needed? Perhaps one might answer that question by saying, "The human body has so much complexity, no one doctor can know everything needed to fix every part." That answer does not explain completely why towns long ago only needed a single "Doc." The human body has not grown more complex in the last few centuries. Perhaps a better answer might go, "The total number of things we now know how to fix in the human body appears to exceed the brain power of any single human to master."

Some historians have suggested that Thomas Jefferson knew everything that humans knew when he was alive. Jefferson certainly studied a significant array of topics in his life, but even he probably never learned everything. In any case, we all understand that today a human life does not last long enough and the brain does not have sufficient neurons, to even come close to mastery of all the skills and information available in this world. So, practitioners of medicine have picked out specific, limited areas (we commonly call them specialties) to master and practice. No doctor today claims to know how to treat the human skin plus all its contents.

In this section, we will introduce you to a long list of medical practice **specialties** and try to link them to parts of the human body, or to categories of treatment methods. Doing that gives you a useful concept of what sort of physician you might want to see for a specific illness or injury. Before we do that, we want to suggest an additional concept.

Medical Investigation 101

The knowledge and methods of treatment that we call medical science appear unlikely to ever stop growing, evolving, and improving. We might expect then that traditional specialties will spawn more subdivisions. We call subdivisions of medical specialties "**sub-specialties**." Consider this example. **Cardiology** designates the specialty of doctors who treat diseases of the heart. In the 1930's Dr. Werner Forssmann demonstrated the possibility of threading a small tube, called a **catheter**, from a vein in his own arm all the way up to his chest ending up inside his own heart. That demonstration launched over a span of decades a long list of diagnostic and treatment procedures Cardiologists can perform. Cardiologists who do these sorts of procedures have created a sub-specialty called **Invasive Cardiology**. In the future as knowledge keeps expanding, we might need sub-sub-specialties, and even sub-sub-sub-specialties. Can you anticipate a problem with such a future for medical care as physicians become more and more focused on just one tiny piece of medical care?

Over the last decade or two, public health experts have come to recognize that medical practitioners appear to make more and more mistakes as they try to cure **diseases** and treat **injuries**. Some of that must come from the fact that so much knowledge has made rapid decision making overwhelming. Also, since medical treatments constantly grow more effective, indeed more powerful, mistakes in using the wrong treatment grow more devastating, even deadly. Some experts have concluded that healthcare practitioners must need more training, more knowledge, to prevent mistakes. More knowledge? We just said too much information appears to have created the problem. We have made the point in this book that anyone electing a career in the healing arts should expect to continue studying and learning endlessly, but will more education prevent mistakes? Does more education stop people from leaving something important off their grocery list or stop people from losing their car keys? Of course, it does not. Human beings make mistakes because the human brain does not work flawlessly. As we learn more about how our brain does the amazing things it can do, we also see the reasons that it makes mistakes.

One category of mistakes in healthcare appears to arise from our current way of moving patients to specialists or sub-specialists to get the proper treatment.

Primary Care physicians see patients who do not have a diagnosis. The **Primary Care** specialist makes a tentative diagnosis and commonly sends the patient on to another specialist. If the first step in the process of getting to the right specialist goes amiss, the patient has a very difficult time getting the correct treatment. The specialist or sub-specialist getting the patient from the Primary Care doctor tends to find a diagnosis within his or her **domain** to explain the patient's problem, perhaps without fully considering all the possible alternative diagnoses that lie in other specialties. Fortunately, many specialists do recognize when a patient came to them by mistake and needs to restart the process, but too many patients fail to recover from an initial mistake in this referral process.

Have you heard the expression "**tipping point**?" The notion of a tipping point describes the process, often seen, in which a long series of gradual changes suddenly brings about a totally new solution or approach to replace an old method of doing things. Since the authors of this book expect our readers to have not yet selected a career, we think it appropriate to warn you that the existing structure of medical specialties that keeps hatching sub-specialties probably is approaching a tipping point. We appear to need a new way to manage medical knowledge and make sure every patient has precisely the right diagnosis before getting directed to an expert in a specific treatment.

How might the future deal with the never-ending growth in medical knowledge and techniques? No one can actually forecast the future, but we might guess that on the other side of this tipping point in medical care, practitioners will stop trying to cram more medical knowledge into their heads and instead rely increasing on what we now call "**artificial intelligence**" to guide them, to double check their conclusions, and even to enhance their procedural skills in healing. Many believe "artificial intelligence" can both reduce mistakes and make procedures more **fault tolerant**. Exactly how that might happen may depend upon you, if indeed you select for yourself a career in the medical arts.

Ray Kurzell, a leader in artificial intelligence research, has coined the term "**hybrid thinking**" to describe the way in which human minds might work with computer systems in the future to enhance human performance in complex fields of work, and even in routine human activities. Humans have unique capabilities to consider ideas outside of what might seem logical while computers never forget details and can search through vast amounts of information without tiring. "Hybrid thinking" represents the promise of combining these two, quite different skillsets to achieve what today we view as impossible. Could we make healthcare immune to errors?

The authors of this book hope, if you do enter a healthcare career, that you will make sure that the future of medical practice retains the highly important aspects of the **doctor-patient relationship** and caring as it changes the things necessary to eliminate errors that do harm. Recognizing that a tipping point lies ahead might indeed make a healthcare career choice even more exciting for people who want their lives to change the world for the better.

In the meantime, doctors decide during their training how they would like to help people by picking one area to study in great depth. They then spend several years learning and practicing what they have learned in just that one area. As we have said, a doctor cannot easily know everything, even within his or her one area of specialization, because discoveries just keep coming. So, all practitioners need **lifelong learning**, plus we must find ways to make that process more consistent and less prone to errors by using evolving concepts like "hybrid thinking."

In this chapter, we hope to introduce you to how today's array of physician specialties might line up to diagnose a patient's condition or assist a patient in their efforts to regain their health. Let's now introduce you to a few medical specialties, just to give you an idea of what categories exist. We cannot begin to cover them all.

A **Gerontologist** specializes on the process of aging and helps patients deal with the ravages of growing old. We start with the Gerontologist because the authors of this book consider that specialty highly important in their personal lives. The Gerontologist works at the opposite end from the **Pediatrician** who, you recognize, specializes in children and their unique diseases.

Should you get seriously injured, which we hope never happens, you might meet a **Trauma Surgeon** in the Emergency Room. A Trauma Surgeon goes through four years of medical school, then does a residency in General Surgery, and finally adds a fellowship in Trauma surgery. Wow! **Medical school** makes one into a doctor. A **residency program** lasting usually three to six years, depending upon the specialty, turns that doctor into a specialist. And then a **fellowship** lasting one to three years makes the specialist into a sub-specialist. Does that sound utterly impossible? If you talk to the individuals who go through these programs, they will tell you they only focus on one day at a time and the pace and excitement of the work leaves little time or energy for counting the days.

Let's get back to your poor body we are pretending to lie badly injured in an emergency room. If you have damaged your chest doing something bad to your lungs or heart a **Cardiothoracic Surgeon** might come to your aid. If instead you banged up your head badly, you would want a **Neurosurgeon** to take your case. On the other hand, if the bones in your leg were broken, an **Orthopedic Surgeon** would take over. Fortunately, you would not be required to figure out which kind of doctor you needed; the **Emergency Physician** (a specialist in emergency care) would figure out for you which specialists you need.

Suppose alternatively you were not feeling well but were not so sick that you needed to go to the emergency room. In that case your Primary Care doctor would sort out what kind of doctor would best solve your issues. Primary Care doctors come from several specialties, specialties that have offices open to patients trying to figure out what is making them not feel well. Those specialties include **Family Practice**, **Internal Medicine**, **Pediatrics**, and often **Gynecology** for female patients.

Let's quickly meet some more specialists. An **Oncologist** takes care of patients who have cancer. A **Radiation Oncologist** sees patients with cancer who need to receive radiation to destroy a cancerous tumor. A **Psychiatrist** works with patients who have depression, anxieties, and other feelings that disrupt their lives. A **Neurologist** sees patients who have issues with their nerves causing symptoms like muscle twinges, numbness, tingling, headaches, or weakness in arms and legs. A **Hematologist** gets called when a patient has abnormal blood. A **Nephrologist** or **Urologist** might help you with problems with your kidneys and urinary bladder.

Medical Investigation 101

What medical specialist do we hardly ever meet in person, but often see on television shows? You probably know a lot about that specialist, the **Pathologist**. Pathologists we call on to figure out what caused someone's death; they appear frequently in mystery stories. You might not appreciate that pathologists constantly help other physicians figure out a diagnosis by studying samples of fluid and tissue sent to them in their laboratories. The life of a Pathologist can prove very challenging and even exciting.

The list of medical specialists goes on and on: **Dermatologist, Otolaryngologist, Obstetrician, Anesthesiologist, Cardiologist, Infectious Disease Specialist, Toxicologist, Podiatrist, Plastic Surgeon, Pulmonologist, Neonatologist**…. but we will leave you to look up the categories that peak your interest.

Now let's pretend you have finished medical school and completed a residency in Family Practice. You have opened an office and patients come to you so you can sort out their symptoms. You can imagine you might feel very lonely having all that responsibility placed on you, but in fact you would recognize that you have all sorts of other medical specialists available to help you out. When physicians ask other physicians for help them, they call that "making a **referral**." Try your hand at figuring out who might help you with these patients: (We put answers at the bottom for you to look at after you work on these cases. Sometimes more than one answer can prove valid.)

(1) A 45-year-old male patient complains of ringing in his ears, a symptom he has had on-and-off for two months. You decide to refer the patient to a specialist. Which one?
(2) An 87-year-old female repeatedly is getting lost in her own neighborhood when she goes for a walk. The woman's daughter brings her to your office for help. Who might have special skills to help this woman?
(3) The mother of a 13-year-old boy brings him to your office. Her son fell off his skateboard while doing ramp jumping in the backyard. He has a swollen, very tender arm. You order an x-ray, which shows a break in the radius bone of the lower arm. What specialist takes care of broken bones?

(4) A 57-year-old man comes to you concerned that he occasionally feels light headed and dizzy. He cannot identify any specific activity that causes this to happen. When you listen to his heart you hear an irregular heart beat and an unusual sloshing sound between the normal beats of the heart. Pick a specialist for him, but don't get distracted by his light headedness symptom.
(5) A 35-year-old female comes to you complaining of pain starting in her right hip and shooting down her right leg. This all started after she moved into a new apartment and lifted lots of furniture and heavy boxes. You find the patient cannot feel sharpness on the skin of the right leg when touched with a pointed probe and she cannot feel the difference between a warm and cold wet gauze touching her right leg. What specialist might she best see?
(6) A mother brings in a 9-year-old girl to see you after the family's pet cat scratched the youngster's face. The mother heard of a disease called "cat scratch fever." You would not treat the child with antibiotics despite the mother's concern, but when you examine the wound you see a surprisingly deep cut on the right cheek below her eye that goes deep enough to require stitches. What specialist would best manage a deep cut on a child's face?

1-Otolaryngologist (aka. Ear Nose & Throat Specialist), 2-Neurologist, 3-Orthopedist, 4-Cardiologist, 5-Neurologist, Neurosurgeon, or Orthopedist could all constitute appropriate referrals for this patient, 6-Plastic Surgeon or Emergency Room Specialist (Emergency Room Specialists suture wounds routinely, although a Plastic Surgeon would prove helpful to revise any scar that might persist after the wound healed).

We may now have your head spinning with the vastness of the types of physicians that exist now, not to mention the possibility of even more types sprouting up in the future. You might find yourself wondering, "How can anyone figure out what path to take with so many roads available?" Please rest assured, you do not need to pick a destination when you start your path to a career. The individual choices you will make in your life along your way

Medical Investigation 101

will always prepare you well for the next choice you will need to make. Right now, we want you to enjoy the view, sort of like enjoying the beauty of a forest without trying to examine every tree.

Investigation 1.2: The Medical Support Team

We have identified many physician specialists who can make people feel better, but doctors can help more people with greater efficiency if they take advantage of support personnel. A **receptionist**, for example, who makes patient appointments obviously makes the process of office-based medicine more efficient. Similarly, **nurses** at various skill levels can make important observations and adjust treatments to improve outcomes. **Technicians** and **therapists** of various types can apply expert skills to gather diagnostic information and carry out treatment programs. The healthcare system probably has as many, or more, categories of non-physician providers as it has kinds of doctors. In fact, today, if we sent all the members of the medical support team on vacation, healthcare would come to a complete halt.

Medicine has traditionally put physicians at the top of the organizational chart as the prime movers of patient care. One can argue that role has shifted over time, and indeed probably needs to continue to shift. In hospitals, doctors normally write orders that others carry out. Increasingly **nurse practitioners** and **physician assistants**, members of the support team, have the authority to write and modify orders on behalf of physicians. The traditional workflow appears to be changing in hospitals in other ways that benefit the patient. Increasingly hospitals are asking physicians to provide information and **objectives** to team members, in addition to prescriptions and orders. When all the members of the care team know the objective of the therapy, they each can add their considerable expertise to make the therapy more effective and more tolerant of errors. Non-physician members of the care team usually spend a great deal more time directly with the patient and thus can make observations the physician may not have had an opportunity to appreciate. When everyone on the care team knows the specific objectives of the treatment, the entire team becomes empowered to share ideas and tailor the therapy to the patient's advantage. The data now exists to show this works!

Patients need the talents of the entire spectrum of medical support team members to make the correct diagnosis and then take the necessary steps to return the patient to good health. If you think only physicians invest years of schooling to learn their skills, you would be mistaken. Many medical support careers require four or more years of college level training. A few roles may still require as little as six months of training, but the amount of schooling needed appears to increase steadily. Beyond the schooling, the proficient members of the health care team have thousands of hours of experience that has honed their clinical expertise. A physician may have a wider breadth of knowledge, but the other members of the team also have extensive, crucial depth of experience in their specific skills that allows them to contribute vital care to the sick and injured.

Below you will see a long list of medical care support roles. This list will not include them all, since new ones seem to constantly emerge as new medical tools and techniques evolve. One of these support roles could describe a career path that would fit your skills, interests, and life goals. As you read the list you might recall the way that one of these professionals helped you or a member of your family.

Medical Support Team Members: **Registered Nurse (RN), Nurse Practitioner, Physician Assistant, Pharmacist, Dental Hygienist, Massage Therapist, Surgical Technician, Phlebotomist, Optometrist, Optician, Licensed Vocational Nurse (LVN), Orthopedic Technician, Respiratory Therapist, Cardiology Technician, Medical Librarian, Radiology Technician, Ultrasound Technician, Occupational Therapist, Medical Records Clerk, Nuclear Medicine Technician, Medical Education Coordinator, Dental Assistant, Speech Therapist, Clinical Psychologist, Audiologist, Physical Therapist**, **Chiropractor,** and more.

You can easily find for yourself information on what each of these jobs involve and how one goes about preparing for such a career. As an example, if you searched for the role of an optometrist you would find this career path focuses specifically on the use of glasses, contact lenses, and even exercises used to correct vision. **Optometrists** overlap some of the services that **Ophthalmologists** provide, but optometrists do not perform eye surgery. We do refer to optometrists using the title "Doctor" because they hold a Doctor of Optometry degree, a degree that differs from the degree Doctor of Medicine.

Physician Assistants get a college degree in a science field before attending a graduate program to become an assistant to a specific specialty of medicine.

They then work under the supervision of a physician seeing patients, doing some therapy, and often assisting in medical procedures. Physician Assistants with experience often seem to work quite independently and have proven a valuable means to provide healthcare to underserved locations in our nation. This use of Physician Assistants has grown now that we have communication capabilities that allow rapid communication of images and conversations that can allow such a physician assistant to become the eyes and hands of a physician physically located miles away.

Nurse Practitioners or Advanced Practice Nurses start by becoming nurses and then take more advanced training in specific areas of medical practice to also work closely with physicians seeing patients and performing therapy appropriate to their skills and experience. They also have played a vital role in extending high quality healthcare to more people across our nation.

Investigation 1.2B: Medical Support Team Referrals

Physicians diagnose the problem causing the patient's complaint often using observation and data generated by other members of the team. The doctor then decides which treatments appear to offer the most help to the patient. Since doctors may not have the time or specific experience necessary to administer many treatments personally, they often **refer** the patient to a member of the **Medical Support Team,** who directly performs the treatments on an appropriate schedule.

Physical Therapists represent a prime example of this support team relationship. Physical Therapists study the anatomy of bones and muscles, along with the use of physical means to restore function. They then use their training, knowledge, and experience to guide patients to a speedy recovery from injury or surgery. Patients with a variety of conditions that can benefit from exercise, stretching, and physical treatments, to include heat, icing, whirlpool, all go to physical therapy. Often, physical therapists actually go to the patient where they live to help them regain strength and movement after an injury or after surgery.

If you have a sore throat with a cough and green phlegm, the doctor might write a prescription for antibiotic pills. Physicians do not keep a supply of all the medicines they prescribe in their office. Instead they send you to a member of the support team who has shelves of medications in a variety of dosage forms. The **Pharmacist** at the drug store knows about potential **interactions** between prescription medicines and has expertise in explaining exactly how the patient can derive the greatest benefit from his or her medications. Pharmacists in the hospital provide a similar vital role in patient care and commonly accompany physicians as they see patients in the hospital to help adjust complex regimens of medications.

Suppose YOU are a Family Practitioner. Read each of these case descriptions and decide what member of the medical support staff you or another practitioner might call upon to help care for the patient. You can see the author's suggested answers at the bottom of this section.

(1) An 11-year-old female fell on her right wrist playing soccer. She felt immediate pain in the area and came to you for evaluation and treatment. An x-ray showed a small fracture, or break, in one of the bones of her wrist. She was placed in a cast for six weeks and the cast removed. Another x-ray showed the fracture healing well. The girl complained that her wrist remained stiff and weak. Who might help with this situation?

(2) A 19-year old male visits your office with a complaint of bad breath. You ask him if he has seen a dentist in the past year and he says, "No." When you peer into his mouth you notice a small amount of redness (erythema) in his gums. You recommend a visit to a dentist as soon as possible. The Dentist examines his teeth and notes small pieces of rotten food between some of his teeth in addition to the erythema in his gum tissue. He finds no cavities. Who would the Dentist refer this patient to for treatment?

(3) A 63-year-old female presents with a complaint that her husband always accuses her of saying "What did you say? He thinks I can't hear him when he speaks, but I think he mumbles." You perform a simple hearing test and observe that her hearing appears diminished in her left ear. You examine her for excess ear wax and find none. At this point you might consider referring this lady for further evaluation, but to whom would she go?

(4) A 62-year-old male has been your patient for many years. About four months ago he suffered a stroke which left him with great difficulty speaking. You believe he might regain some of his speaking skills. Which medical support team member might help him?

(5) You have admitted a 73-year-old male smoker to the hospital with difficulty breathing. Because he smoked for over 50 years you diagnosed emphysema. When you listen to the sounds coming from his lungs using your stethoscope, you hear sounds consistent with pneumonia. Which medical support team member would you call to

help this patient manage expelling the mucous in his lungs while he receives antibiotics for his infection?

(6) A 51-year-old male sees you complaining of intermittent chest pain, which comes on when he exercises significantly. At this moment, his chest does not hurt. Your testing machine is broken, so you refer him to the hospital to have an EKG test. Which member of the hospital support team would most likely perform this test on your patient?

(7) A 39-year-old female has recently returned from a trip to Africa. She complains of intermittent fever and chills, and a lack of appetite. You want to know more about the current diseases occurring in Africa. Which member of the support team could help you find the information so you can know the most likely diseases this patient might have contracted?

(8) A 24-year-old pregnant female wants to determine the sex of her unborn baby. Which member of the support team could perform an ultrasound test that might yield that information?

1-Physical Therapist, 2-Dental hygienist, 3-Audiologist, 4-Speech Therapist, 5-Respiratory Therapist, 6-Cardiology Technician, 7-Medical Librarian, 8-Ultrasound Technician

In the last section, we ended our discussion by deciding that the task of picking a career seems overwhelming. Then we were looking only at the vast number of types of physicians. Now we have added even more careers in which people use their minds and hands every day to make the lives of others richer. If you ask a person working in any one of these career choices how they selected that specific career, you will likely hear them talk about a specific experience or a specific individual that pointed them in the direction they elected. Your personal experiences will probably play that same role, especially when you keep an open mind and take the initiative to ask people about their career when you see them doing something you find interesting.

Investigation 2: Medical Diagnostic Process

2.0 Introduction

2.1 Chief Complaint

2.2 Medical History

2.3 Review of Systems

2.4 Medical Exam

2.5 Difference Diagnosis

2.6 Diagnosis

2.7 SOAP Notes

Investigation

2.0: Introduction: The Medical Diagnostic Process

You have probably discovered how much fun you can have discovering a new word that almost no one else has ever heard before. You can work it into conversation and then explain it to your awed friends, when they look at you dumbfounded. For example, you might say, "I caught my dog this morning practicing **zoopharmacognosy**."

"Doing what?" your friends will ask. "Is that something disgusting?"

"No," you will answer, "Zoopharmacognosy simply means those things animals other than humans do to medicate themselves when they have an injury or illness. Did you think only humans have medicines? No, animals know to use plants, insects, even soils to treat their symptoms. My dog was eating grass this morning, and that seems to cause her to vomit to cure a stomachache. She probably ate something rancid she should not have gone anywhere near. My dog is cute, but not real smart."

We will leave a full review of the fascinating medical practices of the animal kingdom for you to research, because the mission of this section lies solely in providing you a sense of the medical diagnostic process used by humans. Humans most likely got started thousands of years ago in much the same way their non-human ancestors did. They felt badly and by chance found that a certain food or activity allowed them to feel better. Likely they shared those experiences with others, by example or by words, and we feel very confident that medical practice grew from that humble beginning.

As knowledge of medications and treatments grew, specific individuals made the effort to learn all they could about what worked and what did not in order to help others recover from all manner of sickness and injury. Eventually schools came about to teach these skills, and our current concept of doctors, nurses, and medical technicians came into existence.

In the sections that follow we will set forth steps one can take to define the nature of an individual's illness or trauma, identify its cause, seek a treatment, and even document the progress of this process to restore normal, good health. We usually start the process by asking how the patient feels. Feelings, things we cannot see or directly measure, we call **subjective**. We will next collect things (findings or information) that we can measure, touch, and observe, things we call **objective**. Both forms of information have importance.

Experienced physicians can often make a correct diagnosis of a condition simply from talking to the patient over the telephone (using only subjective information). An examination of the patient can add additional clues, but often the appreciation of subtle clues from an examination require the examiner to have unusual skills of observation based on training and experience. (Medical students commonly hear tales of ancient physicians from the Orient who could diagnose diseases of the liver by feeling the patient's pulse. If those stories were ever true, that ability was lost to medical science long ago.")

It makes good sense that one needs a correct **diagnosis** to effectively treat the patient. In this workbook we will stress the importance of getting the correct diagnosis and introduce you to the ways physicians go about getting to that diagnosis. As you work through the lessons you may notice a few instances where we deviate from that path. Physicians sometimes elect to postpone seeking a diagnosis to see how the symptoms evolve. In some instances, physicians start a treatment to see if the response to the treatment will identify the correct diagnosis. We may even see an instance in which a physician guesses a diagnosis and starts treating it because the patient's condition seems too **critical** to even devote time to a thorough physical examination.

We should think of the collection of information from every available source leading to a diagnosis that we have tested for correctness as constituting the **scientific method** in medicine. In addition to this scientific method, we commonly think of medicine as including **art**. What do we mean by the art of medicine? Some would say that the ability of an experienced physician to diagnosis a kidney stone from the way a patient walks into the office constitutes an art. Others might say that the ability to look past an obvious diagnosis and see something more devious or rare as the root cause of a patient's symptoms, we should call an art. All would agree that a physician's ability to sincerely value his or her fellow human being, deeply and personally, in their time of need represents the greatest art in medicine.

Welcome to this introductory presentation of the science and art of medicine.

Investigation 2.1: Chief Complaint

Almost every patient comes to you having a "Chief Complaint". The **Chief Complaint (CC)** is the main problem the patient is concerned about. It may involve pain or a change in the way they feel, or sometimes a simple question or fear about something they heard. Not all patients have a chief complaint; a patient may come to you to have a routine physical exam to assess their current health status. Sometimes patients have more than one complaint, or even a list of complaints. Any complaints after the main, or Chief Complaint, are considered **Secondary Complaints**. Your first challenge is to investigate the Chief Complaint. After you investigate the Chief Complaint you can then investigate any Secondary Complaints.

When investigating the Chief Complaint, you learn as much as possible from the patient. Some patients are better than others describing their complaints. You ask lots of questions to get more information, such as:

- What seems to be the problem?
- When did you first notice this problem?
- What makes it feel better?
- What makes you feel worse?
- Is the problem always in the same place or does it move around?
- What have you tried already before coming here?
- Is the problem constant or does it come and go?
- Is the problem getting better, worse, or staying the same?
- What activities **exacerbate** the problem?
- Does anyone else in your family have this problem?

These are important questions whose answers may guide your investigation. After asking questions you should have a good idea about your patient's **symptoms.** Symptoms provide important clues to the cause of the patient's malady. The answers should tell you if the problem is **acute** or **chronic** and may even set your brain in motion to begin your **differential diagnosis**, a list of possible causes for this complaint. The answers may tell you where to focus your physical examination.

Activity 2.1:

Think about the last time you went to the doctor. Did the nurse or doctor ask you questions like the ones above? On a piece of paper make up a complaint and then write down several questions you would ask a patient to better understand the problem. Remember, medical investigation involves asking lots of questions.

Investigation 2.2: The Medical History

Once your patient has shared their **Chief Complaint**, your **investigation** is about to begin. You must learn everything you can about your patient, starting with their personal **medical history**. You must ask many questions and the patient must answer honestly in order for you to have the best chance of solving their medical mystery.

You need to know their actual age and **gender** because many diseases occur predominately in a specific gender or age group. Some diseases occur mostly in children; others mostly in early adulthood. Still other diseases occur most often later in life. Some diseases occur only in men, while others occur mainly or only in women. Some people look older than their age due to their **lifestyles**. Others look younger than their age because of their **genetic** luck.

You want to explore your patient's current medical status. What other medical problems do they have? Have they recently seen another doctor for the same reason? Were they given **medicines** for this problem by another physician? You need this information to know the patient's assessment of their **current condition** isn't **altered** by the medicine. You would like to know what has worked or not worked in the past if the patient has been treated for a similar condition before. You don't want to give them more of the same medicine and cause an **overdose**. Finally, it would be helpful to know if another recent condition relates to the patient's current **Chief Complaint**; is the problem **acute** or **sub-acute**?

Now that you understand the patient's current status, delving into their medical history can provide additional useful information. What diseases in their past might affect their health today or in the future? Have they undergone treatments having **long-term side effects**? Do they **bleed** easily? Have they ever had **surgery**?

Finally, don't forget to ask about their "family history". Your awareness of diseases such as diabetes and cancer in other members of your patient's family is vital. These diseases can increase the risk of occurrence in your patient as well.

Is there anything else you should know about? Don't allow your patient to decide what is important; you must decide! Your patient may not know how one disease affects another. But you understand because of your medical training and experience treating other patients as you developed your medical "**art**" and '**judgment**".

Look at the two sample patients on the following pages. They provide basic information about the patients' current complaints and their medical histories. There may be more questions you wish to ask to learn more about things in their history that might be important in evaluating their current health status.

Activity 2.2.: Noting important details in the medical history

It is important to make note of any positive medical history findings. Any positive findings in the medical history questionnaire should be confirmed with the patient. For example, "In the medical history you wrote that you have had diabetes for 5 years; is this correct?"

Examine the medical histories of Patients 1 and 2 below. Make a mental note of all positive factors in each patient's medical history. After you have identified all of the positives, you can role play if you have a partner. Take turns being the doctor. Interview your patient about the positives in their medical history. Ask questions about the positives to get more information. Do you understand why doctors ask so many questions?

Patient 1:

Medical History

Patient Name: use your name or a pseudo-name of your choice

Age: 43 **Birthdate:** your birthday   **Gender:** male

Occupation: jack hammer operator

Chief Complaint: numbness and tingling in fingers and hands, weakness in hands and arms

Current Medicines:

1. aspirin 325 mg as needed for headaches and hand pain

2. Advair® steroid inhaler

Past Medical Conditions:

1. asthma since childhood

Last Medical Evaluation: 8 years ago

Childhood Illnesses:

1. chicken pox
2. measles
3. mumps

Past Medical History

1. asthma since childhood
2. allergies to cat dander, grasses and pollens
3. broken left wrist 11 years ago

Family Medical History

mother: type 2 diabetes

father: heart condition

siblings: sister has type 1 diabetes

Surgical History

tonsillectomy age 4

appendectomy age 14

wisdom teeth removed (4) age 23

Medical Investigation 101

Patient 2:

Medical History

Patient Name: use your name or a pseudo-name of your choice

Age: 61 **Birthdate:** your birthdate   **Gender:**   female

Occupation: outside sales

Chief Complaint: headaches and occasional palpitations in chest

Current Medicines: aspirin for headaches, Maalox for stomach upset, estrogen

Past Medical Conditions: stomach ulcer treated 10 years ago

Last medical Evaluation: 5 years ago

Childhood Illnesses: strep throat, pink eye, roseola

Past Medical History

1. Stomach ulcer treated 10 years ago
2. 2 children by C-section many years ago

Family Medical History

Mother: uterine cancer

Father: hypertension and heart condition

Siblings: older brother has heart condition and hypertension

Surgical History

Cataract left eye 2 years ago

C- Section 39 and 41 years ago

Hysterectomy age 54

Investigation 2.3: Review of Systems

Let's take a moment to review what we have accomplished so far. Your patient has told you about their current complaint. You now need to learn about their overall health; that means any medical condition for which they have been treated in the past. You need to know what medicines they take and what types of surgery they may have undergone previously. You also want to know what diseases their parents had, just in case the disease is passed on to the next generation. Put all that information together in a way that the **positives** do not get forgotten. You should carefully review the details of their past medical history with the patient to ensure they have not omitted important events that might change the treatment plan you would recommend.

Doctors classify medical facts as either positives or negatives. **Positive** means yes, that condition or event happened, while **Negative** means no, that condition or event did not occur. Positive findings usually have the greatest value, but careful physicians always document a summary of negative findings as well, because negative findings prove valuable to rule out conditions in a thorough **differential diagnosis**.

As you discuss his or her medical history with your patient, you create the patient's **chart**. The chart is the record about that patient. Every patient has a chart. It allows you, the doctor, to quickly see what you know about your patient when they come back the next time for **follow-up** or a new problem. No doctor can remember every detail about every patient they have ever seen. You have the patient's chart to review what happened in the past so you can see how that patient's health changes over time.

Healthcare providers commonly use abbreviations when they write notes about their patients, as you may do when you take Cornell notes. They use abbreviations to save time. When you have ten patients waiting to see you and you are late to a meeting at the hospital, you understand the lure of abbreviating. Abbreviations, unfortunately, can and have led to mistakes in healthcare. Hospitals have outlawed many abbreviations and created lists of acceptable ones that will not lead to misunderstanding. Have you ever

Medical Investigation 101

wondered later what that abbreviation you wrote while taking notes referred to? Taking care of the health of real human beings requires a special effort to keep accurate and clear records; so, abbreviations have become an issue.

Investigation 2.4: Medical Examination

Now that you have information about the patient's medical history and know why they came to see you today, you are now ready to touch the patient. I know what some of you are thinking: Really, do I have to touch them?

Healthcare practitioners think of the human body as consisting of a number of physiological systems: circulatory, respiratory, digestive, nervous, musculoskeletal, endocrine, urinary, immunologic, and integument. Physicians pride themselves on their ability to examine all of these systems when they evaluate a new chief complaint. When a patient returns for further evaluation of an existing condition, the examiner may not conduct such a thorough evaluation of every system. However, physicians have often embarrassed themselves by not repeating a thorough examination before referring a patient they have failed to diagnose after several visits. They are embarrassed because the new doctor does a thorough examination and finds obvious clues to the correct diagnosis the original physician would have found if he or she had repeated a complete examination.

The process of examining a patient makes use of your natural senses. The first tool you use to examine your patient is your eyes. You look at your patient's skin carefully for signs of infection or skin abnormalities such as a rash, bumps, swelling, redness, or an obvious wound or deformity. You look at their eyes to see if they are clear and looking back at you. You look to see if all the parts are present, such as two ears, two eyes, two arms, and two legs. Absence of one of these indicates a major medical event occurred in their past. You also look for scars that indicate a past injury or surgery. Finally, watching them walk can provide evidence of injury, illness, or deformity.

We also conduct the exam with our ears, such as **auscultation** of the abdomen and back. Did you know that doctors can learn to tell the condition of your liver and lungs by listening carefully as they thump with this technique?

Medical Investigation 101

The sense of touch makes our hands an important tool for examining patients. We can feel lumps that should not exist. We can feel the strength of muscles. We can push on the abdomen and feel the edge of an enlarged liver or **elicit** pain from an injured organ. We can touch the patient and ask if they feel that touch or feel tingling or prickles that suggest damage to peripheral nerves (termed **paresthesia**). We can also tap on the abdomen or chest to see if that tapping produces the expected hollow sound, or a dullness suggestive of something abnormal.

Beyond our built-in senses, the **stethoscope** represents the most **ubiquitous** tool for examining patients. The stethoscope is very valuable because it can be used to examine so many areas in the body. For example, you know you can hear your heartbeat with a stethoscope; you can also hear heart problems. You can hear the pulsing of arteries in your neck, arms, and legs and even the sounds movement in your intestines as food moves. The stethoscope can also be used with a **sphygmomanometer** to measure your blood pressure. Can you say sphygmomanometer three times really fast? I can't. But it's a really important tool.

Another important tool is the **reflex hammer**. It's a hammer because you hit people with it. But you have to hit them in the right places and not too hard. This hammer is used to detect the presence or absence of your reflexes. Reflexes are reactions that do not require your brain to respond. You have reflexes that can be detected using the hammer in your arms and legs. You also have what is called a **plantar reflex** on the bottom of your foot. It is interesting to test this reflex; you rub the skinny end of the hammer along the outer plantar foot surface. If the big toe points upward, the patient may have a brain abnormality on the opposite side; that would be called a **positive Babinski sign**.

Historically, some physicians became famous because they had an ability to examine patients so keenly that they almost never failed to make a correct diagnosis simply from the patient's history and examination findings. Perhaps to allow all physicians to perform at that level, we now have more sophisticated tools that take us far beyond our own senses in the search for the correct diagnosis. We use these additional tests to add to the information from the physical examination. Some of these tools we can bring into the physician's office, while others live in hospitals because of the size or cost of those tools.

Some parts of the body cannot be examined by looking with your eyes, or touching with your hands, or even using a simple instrument. For example, examining the condition of the blood requires taking a little blood from the patient and having it analyzed. It is amazing how much we can learn about a patient by having their blood analyzed. For years patients have endured having vial after vial of blood taken from them, enough to feed a vampire. Recently, technology has been developed that allows blood to be completely analyzed using only a single drop of blood. This is great news for patients! And remember, doctors are sometimes patients, too.

Sometimes we need to look inside the patient as part of our investigation. But we don't usually need to cut them open to look inside. If we want to see the condition of bones, we can order an **x-ray**. If we need to better examine **tissue** such as **muscle, tendons** and **ligaments** we can order an **MRI (**magnetic resonance imaging). To further evaluate the heart, arteries and veins, or even the growth of a fetus we can utilize **ultrasound.**

Activity 204: Testing the Plantar Response. Find a partner. Take off your shoes and socks. Have your partner sit on a table or desk with their feet hanging in a relaxed manner. Using a neurological hammer if you have one, or the eraser end of a pencil, rub the eraser along the outside surface of the bottom of your partner's feet, one foot, then the other foot. You should observe the big toe move downward without any effort from your partner.

If you check on an infant you need to know that it is normal for very young children to have a positive test, or upward movement of the big toe. In older children and adults, the big toe should move downward.

Investigation 2.5: Differential Diagnosis

Now that you have taken a thorough medical history and examined your patient, you are ready to start analyzing what you have learned in your investigation and start finding possible answers. You may have ordered one or more preliminary tests to assist you further, but mentally you have been formulating opinions on what might be causing the patient's symptoms.

Doctors try to determine all of the known conditions that are capable of causing the symptoms revealed by the patient and your examination. This list of possibilities is known in medical investigation as the "**Differential Diagnosis**", or DDx. If there is any doubt about the most likely cause, the physician will start "**ruling out**" life threatening conditions first. One set of symptoms can cause you to develop a Differential Diagnosis having fifteen or more suspects. Just like a police lineup, you see if the symptoms match the suspect disease; if not, you might remove it from the list or give it a lower **priority** for further evaluation.

For example, here is a potential Differential Diagnosis for a complaint of "Chest Pain" according to the Cleveland Clinic[1], a very well respected medical center:

Cardiac causes of chest pain are: ischemia (due to blockages - including both stable and unstable angina and acute heart attack and coronary artery spasm), pericarditis (inflammation of the sack around the heart), myocarditis (inflammation of the heart), cardiomyopathy (heart failure) and rarer causes such as coronary artery dissection, acute rupture of the heart and valves and infections of the pericardium.

Pulmonary (lung) causes include: pneumonia, pulmonary embolus, pneumothorax, pleuritis and bleb rupture.

Other potential causes are: aortic dissection, back and spine problems and musculoskeletal (muscle strain, rib fracture, etc.).

Psychological causes of chest pain are: common and include panic attacks, anxiety, stress and mental duress.

Above is a list of over twenty possible causes of chest pain. So sometimes it can take a while for the physician to find the actual cause of the pain. Making a Differential Diagnosis requires serious thinking and often requires getting help from medical books and reputable internet sources, especially when analyzing problems you have not experienced treating before. There are also medical specialists, physicians with more experience evaluating or treating that particular set of symptoms, to which you can consult and refer your difficult to diagnose patients.

1. http://my.clevelandclinic.org/services/heart/disorders/coronary-artery-disease/causes-chest-pains

Investigation 2.6: The Diagnosis

The practice of medicine starts with making the right **diagnosis.** If you don't make the correct diagnosis your patient will suffer because your misdirected treatment will not work; time wasted on the wrong treatment may allow your patient's condition to worsen. So, you have a tremendous responsibility in medical practice to make the correct diagnosis.

In order to make the correct diagnosis you, as the doctor, must consider all of the possible causes for the patient's symptoms. The task can prove difficult because many diseases or injuries can have very similar **symptoms**. You must solve the medical mystery, just as the crime scene investigator must solve the crime mystery. Sometimes in the case of a crime the detective arrests the wrong person and a court may convict an innocent person, all because the investigator left the real criminal off the suspect list. In medicine, if you don't have the cause of your patient's disease in your **differential diagnosis**, you may make an incorrect diagnosis and sentence your patient to unnecessary pain, disability, or even death.

When patients come to you for advice or treatment, their **chief complaint** will usually relate to not feeling well or suffering an **injury**. The patient tells you their **symptoms**; your analysis of their symptoms and test results helps you form your differential diagnosis. When you analyze this list of possible causes of the symptoms, you think about which of their symptoms might *not* fit with the diagnoses on your list. You try to **rule-out** the possible diagnoses one-by-one by asking more questions, examining the patient more carefully, or doing additional laboratory tests until only one diagnosis remains, the correct one. Virtually every diagnosis you make as a physician will fall into one of three categories: **Infection, Injury,** or **Genetic Disorder**.

When we think of an **illness**, an infection probably jumps first into our minds. But an illness can also result from an injury or even a genetic origin. As the treating physician it makes sense to first determine whether your patient's illness arises from an infection. Genetic disorders and injuries do not spread to the people around you. However, we call many infections **communicable** because they can easily spread to others. Diagnosing communicable diseases quickly may keep an infection from spreading through your entire neighborhood or beyond. Focus first on the possibility of an infection.

You can normally diagnose acute injuries more easily. If your patient tells you that yesterday he fell off his skateboard and now his wrist is swollen and painful, you already know with some certainty that the fall injured his wrist. But your differential diagnosis should include both a fracture and a sprain, and perhaps even a couple very rare causes of wrist swelling and pain, because you don't yet know the diagnosis with certainty. Sometimes patients don't come to you until several days or even weeks have passed since their injury. Sub-acute injuries, injuries that do not seem too bad at first, can make your diagnostic challenge much more difficult. Think about the last time you had an injury. Did you use the injured part right away? Probably not. People normally protect an injured area from movement or stress so it will not hurt. When we protect our injured area we might then overuse another part of our body. This effort to protect can cause pain in the overused area that wasn't injured originally. So be careful when you diagnose the cause of a sub-acute injury to make sure you find the primary site of injury.

Genetic disorders are **deformities** or diseases that parents carry and pass on unknowingly to their children. Some of these disorders are passed on by only one parent, while others require the condition to be carried by both parents. Some genetic disorders present at birth, such as a **cleft palate**, while others may not show symptoms until later years, like **epilepsy**.

Use your **differential diagnoses** list to eliminate possibilities one-by-one until you have only the correct diagnosis left. In reality doctors often cannot eliminate with certainty all but one potential cause. In that case, you must use your **judgment** to go ahead and treat the injury or illness despite the uncertainty. That decision makes sense if the treatment has little chance of harming your patient, or if the treatment response proves your uncertain diagnosis correct. Some call these judgment decisions in the face of uncertainty the **"Art"** of Medicine. If medical care was provided based only on science, no one would receive treatment without a proven diagnosis, and patients would suffer from long delays. You, as a doctor, must use your judgment in analyzing

Medical Investigation 101

all available information to decide on a treatment plan while still searching for new information and options. That aspect of the **"Art"** requires years to develop.

Never forget: Patients put their trust in you, the physician, to do your best to diagnose and treat their injuries and illnesses to the best of your ability. It is a sacred responsibility that should never be taken lightly.

The lessons in this text will challenge you to solve medical mysteries for the benefit of your patients. You will have an opportunity to practice and develop your skills of evaluation, analysis, and diagnosis. Don't forget to make a thorough Differential Diagnosis for each case you investigate so that you can consider all of the possible causes. The ability to work through a list of options to find the best solution will serve you well in solving cases from this book as well as solving the crises in your own life. We are confident you are up to the challenge.

Before you begin solving the medical investigations to follow, let's practice classifying diagnoses. Next you will find an activity to help you think about how to classify the challenges you will encounter later.

One of the initial challenges you have as a physician is to classify your patient's chief complaint. In this activity you will practice classifying disorders into their category. Number on your paper from 1 to 20. Study each condition and write on your paper whether you think it is caused by infection, injury, or genetic occurrence.

Activity 2.6

Legend: Caused by Infection = **INF** Caused by Injury = **INJ** Genetic cause = **GEN**

1. Natural Red Hair
2. Sprained Ankle after soccer game
3. Stomach ache after eating potato salad at picnic
4. Pimples on face
5. Concussion after football game
6. Down Syndrome
7. Chicken Pox
8. Infected ingrown toenail
9. Cystic Fibrosis
10. Blue Eyes
11. Fractured wrist after a fall
12. Muscular Dystrophy
13. Fractured Pelvis after a car accident
14. Polio
15. Infant born with six toes on each foot
16. Ebola
17. Quadriplegic after fall from roof
18. Small Pox
19. 2nd degree burns after a fire
20. Tuberculosis

How many did you know? If you got them all correct you may already be a candidate for medical school. Correct answers at the end of Investigation 2.7.

Investigation 2.7: Soap Notes

Commonly physicians use **SOAP** Notes to track a patient's progress on subsequent visits to their office. SOAP notes represent an organizational tool for information about the patient's complaints, examination findings and test results, professional opinions on cause, and assessment or treatment plan going forward. SOAP, an acronym, stands for Subjective, Objective, Assessment, and Plan.

You took a complete history and examination during the patient's first visit to your office. You do not need to repeat the process every time you see this patient. Now, when they return to see you, you need only to add new observations and new patient experiences related to the patient's original complaint.

Each SOAP note has a title taken from a list of the patient's problems. Today you are seeing a patient with only one problem on her Problem List, "Trauma to left wrist." If the patient presents with a new problem that you believe has no relationship to the original complaint, you would add that complaint to the patient's problem list and initiate a new series of SOAP notes under that title to track the new problem. Some physicians number their problem list and attach the appropriate number to each SOAP note instead of writing out a title. When treatment gets rid of a problem the physician joyfully strikes that problem off the list, usually adding the date on that line to document the triumph.

S - Subjective findings convey the patient's symptoms and experience exactly as they tell you about it. You were not there so you are documenting the patient's description. Subjective information helps you, but patient perceptions may not always prove accurate. You must weigh the subjective information against the objective information that you will record in the next section of the SOAP note.

When writing SOAP notes physicians commonly use abbreviations to save time. They use standardized abbreviations that other health professionals will easily recognize to avoid misunderstanding. Working efficiently benefits more patients, so the use of abbreviations represents a patient benefit when used properly.

O - Objective findings list the results of your examination or laboratory tests. Skin erythema might go on the objective findings list; you see the redness of the skin. Edema constitutes an objective finding; you can measure swelling of the ankle. An elevated white cell count would go on the objective finding list; it reports the outcome of a laboratory test. An X-Ray represents objective information; it shows anatomical findings relevant to the patient's complaint. You may find yourself wanting to add your opinion or a supposition in this part of the note, but save that for the next section.

A - Assessment records your professional opinions on the status of this problem. The assessment is based on the subjective information provided by the patient and your objective findings from your observations and test results. Your assessment may conclude that the solution to this problem remains unknown; perhaps the answer awaits results from tests not yet performed. Most importantly, you will return to the assessment when this patient returns again to your office. The assessment will remind you where you left off in your quest to solve this investigation.

P - Plan summarizes the treatments or tests you are recommending at this visit. If you prescribe an antibiotic to treat a suspected or documented bacterial infection, write that in the plan. If you recommend a test, such as an X-Ray or blood test, you list that in the plan. A prescription for physical therapy or an ultrasound goes into the plan.

Before the patient's next visit to your office your staff will receive the results of any tests that you have ordered. They will bring any abnormal findings to your attention for immediate consideration, and all results will go into the objective findings of the next SOAP note that you write.

SOAP notes represent a systematic method of keeping you organized on the current issues (or problems) in each patient's care. With so many patients in your medical practice, you cannot reliably remember everything that is going on with each patient. You need a system to avoid mistakes. SOAP provides you that organizational tool that saves you time and avoids missing important clues to the right diagnosis and treatment. Every patient wants to feel confident that you have complete control of their care; SOAP notes allow you to quickly refresh your memory so that when you walk into that examination room you give each patient the level of care they expect and deserve.

Now we will look at a sample of a SOAP note on a hypothetical patient. Below each entry you will find a translation of the abbreviations a physician would use to write efficiently the SOAP notes.

S: 45 Y.O. female C/O pain in L wrist of 3 wks duration, not resolving. Hit wrist kitchen counter, pain hours later. She self Txd c̄ ASA TID x 5 days w/o resolution or improvement.

Translation: A 45 year-old female is complaining of pain in her left wrist of three weeks duration that is not getting better. She recalls hitting her wrist on the kitchen counter but did not experience pain until several hours later. She self-treated with aspirin three times per day for five days without the pain improving or going away.

O: 2+/4 **edema** L wrist; 0/4 edema R wrist

2+/4 pain L wrist **extension** palmer, 0/4 pain dorsal

1+/4 pain wrist **flexion** on palmer, 0/4 pain dorsal

No erythema or induration

Translation:

Moderate soft tissue swelling of the left wrist; no swelling on the right wrist.

Moderate pain in the left wrist on outwardly extending the wrist felt on the palm side of hand; no pain felt on the wrist of the back side of the hand.

Mild Pain felt on the palm side of the wrist moving the moving wrist into flexion (curled forward); no pain on the back of the wrist.

No redness or thickening of the skin to suggest chronic swelling.

A: Mod Sprain L Wrist

          R/O fracture

Translation: Moderate sprain left wrist; rule-out fracture of a bone.

P: 1. Wrist splint – remove for bathing only

        2. Rx: X-ray L wrist

        3. Rx: Ibuprofen 800mg/TID 5 days c food

        4. Ret 1 wk eval progress

        5. Call pt c X-ray results

Translation:

1. Patient to wear a wrist splint except when bathing
2. Prescription: X-ray Left wrist
3. Prescription: Ibuprofen 800mg Three Times per Day with food
4. Return in one week to evaluate progress
5. Call patient with X-ray results

When the patient returns you can quickly refer to the assessment and plan to remind yourself where you left off with this patient and to know exactly what you are looking for at this upcoming visit. If you had seen 200 patients during the week, without SOAP notes you probably would not recall all the details of her problem and progress.

Think about the times you have been to the doctor to check on your progress in recovering from a sickness or injury. Did your doctor know why you were there? Please remember that patients want to feel that you care about them personally. Poor organization can destroy your patient's confidence in you in the blink of an eye. SOAP notes keep you organized, save you time, and help you always appear in control and well informed about your patients' problems.

Food for thought. Elsewhere in this book you will find comments on the future of medicine requiring new ways to manage the vast amount of information we call medical science. Human memory, long seen as the mainstay of medical practice, can no longer fulfill our expectations for consistent accuracy, day and night, when human lives depend on the right diagnosis and treatment. The heroes and heroines of modern medicine will increasingly become those individuals who figure out work methods by which every healthcare professional can perform at the level of the best experts in that area. Dr. Lawrence Weed, M.D., had that vision of medical practice even in 1968, when he published an article describing the problem-oriented medical record. The SOAP note came from that publication. Weed lectured often during his career about the fact that patient's commonly die in the hospital on the wrong service, meaning their primary doctor, trained in one specialty, did not recognize and treat a complication much better understood in another specialty. Weed believed strongly that computer technology could bridge this knowledge gap and provide greater patient safety. Most would argue Weed's dream has not yet been fulfilled, but the need for others with his vision has never been greater.

ANSWERS FOR ACTIVITY 2.6

1. GEN	8. INF	15. GEN
2. INJ	9. GEN	16. INF
3. INF	10. GEN	17. INJ
4. INF	11. INJ	18. INF
5. INJ	12. GEN	19. INJ
6. GEN	13. INJ	20. INF
7. INF	14. INF	

Investigation 3.1

3.1A: Breathing Difficulty

3.1B: Pulmonary Embolism

Investigation 3.1A: Breathing Difficulty

"Good morning, Doctor" says Betsy, an 18-year-old female, speaking with difficulty. You notice she is sitting up very straight on your **examination table** and appears **agitated**. "I'm having a lot of trouble breathing. I just can't get enough air, and I'm scared." Betsy is depending on you to figure out why she feels so **distressed.**

As you **listen and observe** Betsy, you see that she is working very hard to breathe. You see the muscles in her neck **contracting** as she tries to take in more air. You count the number of times she breathes in 30 seconds and determine she is breathing in and out more than 30 times a minute, whereas a normal rate is about 18 breaths per minute. During this time of careful observation, you see a tightly wrapped **elastic** bandage covering Betsy's left calf, ankle, and half of her foot.

When you ask Betsy how long she has felt this way, she tells you she was fine last night, but woke up this morning feeling this way. She states she has never felt like this before, and has not been sick recently, but **sprained** her left ankle three days ago playing soccer.

You have enough information to begin your examination. Observation has already demonstrated that Betsy is breathing rapidly. You take out your **stethoscope** and first listen to her lungs because her main complaint is difficulty breathing. You hear normal **breath sounds** in both lungs. Moving the stethoscope to the area of the heart, you hear a very rapid heart rate of 115 beats per minute; a normal rate would fall between 60 and 80 beats per minute. Finally, you perform one more test that will provide helpful information. Your nurse attaches the pulse **oximeter** to Betsy's right index finger and reveals her **oxygen saturation** is 76%; a normal oxygen saturation registers between 95% and 100%.

Doctors commonly begin their assessment of any patient by classifying the urgency of the patient's medical problem. If the symptoms came on suddenly we call the condition a**cute.** If the symptoms have existed for weeks or months we classify the condition as **chronic.** If the symptoms are growing worse by the minute we have an **emergency** and need to treat that condition quickly. If the patient's symptoms appear stable, not an emergency, we can take more time for assessment without placing the patient's health in jeopardy.

Doctors also try to determine all of the known conditions that are capable of causing the symptoms the patient reports and the examination reveals. This list of possibilities is known in medical investigation as the "**Differential Diagnosis**". If the physician has any doubt about the most likely cause, he or she will start "**ruling out**" life threatening conditions first. For the patient described above at least fifteen different conditions could potentially cause her breathing difficulty.

Here is a Differential Diagnosis for Patient Betsy:

Pneumonia	Chronic Obstructive Pulmonary Disease	Tuberculosis
	Pulmonary Hypertension	Choking	Epiglottitis
	Asthma	Heart Failure
Pulmonary Embolus	Chest Wall Compression
Anxiety	Hiatal Hernia	Obesity	Altitude Sickness	Allergic Reaction

This means that you, Betsy's new doctor, must mentally check off whether each of these medical conditions could be the cause of Betsy's breathing difficulty. Some are easy to rule out, such as choking and altitude sickness. Others you can rule out because they do not fit the pattern of Betsy's complaint and what you found in your examination. Finally, a few conditions are left on your list for you to evaluate by additional examination or medical tests.

Investigation 3.1B: Pulmonary Embolism

In your role as a busy Family Doctor your patients come to you for many medical problems. Many are within your ability to diagnose and treat confidently using your knowledge and the limited medical equipment in your office. To make the correct diagnosis may require specialized tests, some of which can only be performed in a hospital. Sometimes a problem is complicated enough that you would best serve the patient by sending them to a physician specializing in that area of the body or that particular medical condition. Betsy may well be one of those patients.

One of the conditions that should have worked its way up to near the top of your differential diagnosis is **pulmonary embolism**. Betsy has an acute problem, as she felt fine the day before presenting with difficulty breathing. The tightly wrapped ankle and history of recent injury are clues to the potential origin of her current problem.

So, what is a pulmonary embolism and how does it happen? The word **pulmonary** is the medical word referring to the lung. An **embolism** is an obstruction, or blockage, of an artery by an air bubble, fat or a **blood clot**; in Betsy's case a blood clot (the embolus) most likely caused her embolism. A blood clot is a clump of blood cells that have stuck together.

It is possible that the bleeding that occurred internally when Betsy sprained her ankle resulted in some of the blood cells clumping together as the body tried to heal her ankle injury. If the clot broke loose inside the vein taking blood back to the **central circulation** (heart and lungs), it is possible for the embolus to get stuck in a lung and block circulation through part of that lung. That would make it difficult for Betsy to get enough oxygen into her circulation because air is going to portions of the lung that have no blood flow; that would cause Betsy to have a rapid rate of breathing as she tried harder and harder to get more oxygen into her circulation. A blockage in the lung reduces **air exchange** and causes the heart to beat more rapidly as cells throughout the body cry out for more oxygen. Would you consider this a potential emergency situation?

As a Family Doctor you realize this patient needs immediate evaluation, including several tests to confirm the diagnosis. If your hunch proves correct, Betsy will require intensive treatment that a specialist in lung diseases can best provide. You would probably call on a Pulmonologist and have him or her meet Betsy at the hospital, where she would be admitted as a patient.

Treatment of the blood clot might include **thrombolytic** drugs designed to break up the blood clot. That method of treatment is only available for a limited time following the onset of symptoms, so Betsy needs to get to the hospital right away. Following the acute treatment Betsy might be placed on an **anticoagulant** drug, a medicine that lessens the blood's ability to clot. It would be important that Betsy be careful in her lifestyle so she wouldn't accidentally injure herself in a way that might cause her to bleed to death.

In this case you made a good decision to refer Betsy to the pulmonologist so that she could be admitted to the hospital. The final diagnosis was Pulmonary Embolism. The pulmonologist was able to dissolve the clot using a thrombolytic medicine. Betsy was sent home after a few days and continues on anticoagulant medicine.

What would have happened if Betsy had developed pulmonary **emboli** (the plural of embolus) in both lungs? That circumstance probably would not have had such a happy outcome.

Investigation 3.2

3.2A: Abdominal Pain

3.2B: Microbes

Investigation 3.2A: Abdominal Pain

Introduction:

Patients commonly come to see their physician complaining of **abdominal pain**. We often call the body cavity below our rib cage our "stomach." Actually, the **abdominal cavity** contains several important organs in addition to the actual stomach. Because many of these organs work together to turn our food into energy and raw materials for sustaining life, malfunction of any organ in this cavity appears to invoke similar **symptoms**. **Diagnosing** the exact cause of illness can prove quite challenging. You, as the treating physician, must look for subtle details in the symptoms in order to reduce your differential diagnosis to a manageable list.

Often the patient has pain in a specific region of the **abdomen** so that we can focus our attention on the organ located there. Physicians commonly divide the abdomen into four quadrants with each **quadrant** containing a different list of organs. This four-zone map of the abdomen helps us think about what organs and other structures are located inside the painful area and thus guides us to possible causes of the illness. Look at the chart and learn which structures are located in each quadrant.

> **RUQ** = **right upper quadrant** containing liver, right kidney, gall bladder, and parts of colon and pancreas.
> **LUQ** = **left upper quadrant** containing stomach, left kidney, spleen, and parts of colon and pancreas.
> **RLQ** = **right lower quadrant** containing appendix, small intestine, major artery and vein to right leg, and parts of ureter and colon.
> **LLQ** = **left lower quadrant** containing major artery and vein to left leg and parts of colon, small intestine, and ureter.

Medical Investigation 101

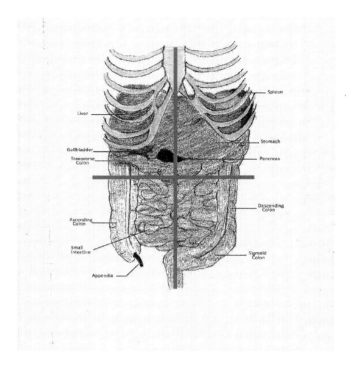

Remember the patient's right side sits on your left side when you face that patient, as if you were looking at yourself in the mirror. The patient's heart lies on the right as you see the patient, even though it is located on their left side. The same principle applies to the organs located in the abdomen.

It is almost time to call it a day and prepare for the weekend as you finish up your shift in the local emergency room of your small rural-community hospital. You have only one more patient to see before you begin two days of relaxation with your family. When you pull back the curtain you find a thirteen-year-old girl doubled over in pain, accompanied by a very worried mother. The girl is crying so you ask the mother what has happened.

Chief Complaint:

The mother, Mrs. Nguyen, reports that earlier today her daughter complained of a stomach ache. The stomach ache grew worse as the day progressed. She thinks maybe something her daughter Crystal ate is causing the problem. The mother reports her daughter has been healthy in the past. The daughter painfully confirms she felt fine yesterday and in the previous weeks. Last night she had dinner with friends at a local fast-food restaurant before going with them to see a movie. None of her friends seem to have any stomach problems.

The girl describes her pain as alternating in intensity between 7/10 and 10/10 since this morning, pointing to the lower right portion of her abdomen near her **umbilicus** and running her hand around to her right side as the area of concern. She has felt nauseated most of the day and she threw up twice. She feels bloated, has no appetite, and had chills and then sweating a few hours ago. She feels as though she needs to pass gas but cannot. The pain increases if she gets up to walk or makes any sudden movement.

Review of Systems:

    Height = 64 inches   Weight = 108 pounds

    No history of allergies

    Vaccinations up to date

    No currents medications

    No previous surgeries

    Chief Complaint: Abdominal Pain

Medical Investigation 101

Examination:

You begin your exam with Crystal sitting on the side of the **gurney**:
- Height and weight deferred due to patient's discomfort on standing.
- Temperature: 101.9 F.
- **Pulse**: 92 bpm
- **Respirations**: 22 / minute
- Heart: **sinus rhythm**
- Lungs: Clear
- A slight yellowish color of her eye **sclera** and skin is noted.

You then ask Crystal to lie back in a **supine** position on the exam table so you can perform a more thorough examination of her abdominal area. Abdominal exam findings:

- **Abdominal distention** is noted. **Bowel sounds** are absent.
- **Rebound tenderness** is elicited in the right lower quadrant.

Differential Diagnosis:

Many things can cause abdominal pain, so the differential diagnosis can be extensive:

Symptoms:

	Jaundice	Abdominal Pain	Bloating	Weight Loss	Loss of Appetite	Stool Change	Urine Dark	Acute/ Chronic	Nausea	Fever	New Diabetes	Pain Radiates
Acute Pancreatitis		x	x	x	x			A	x	x	x	x
Cholangitis	x	x		x	x	x	x	A	x	x	x	x
Peptic Ulcer Disease		x		x	x	x	x	C	x	x		x
Cholecystitis	x	x		x	x	x	x	AC	x	x	x	x
Food Poisoning	x		x		x	x		A	x	x		x
Gastric Cancer	x	x	x	x	x	x		C	x	x		x
Pancreatic Cancer	x	x	x	x	x	x	x	C	x	x	x	x
Hepatoma	x	x		x	x	x	x	C	x	x		x
Appendicitis	x	x	x		x	x		A	x	x		x
Intestinal Ischemia		x	x	x	x	x	x	A	x	x		
Abdominal Aortic Aneurysm		x		x				C	x	x		x
Chronic Pancreatitis	x			x		x	x	C	x		x	x
Patient Crystal												

You might have noticed that many of the symptoms for each illness listed in the (partial) differential diagnosis chart are the same. When attempting to eliminate conditions from the list you might look at whether a condition is **acute** or **chronic**. But always remember, chronic conditions had their beginnings as an acute condition. So that criteria may not help.

Look more closely at **subtle** differences in symptoms, such as where in the abdomen the patient located the discomfort, or what type of changes she reports related to her stools, to help focus your differential diagnosis.

The chart below can help you use the information from your examination of the patient's abdomen. You pressed on her abdomen and then quickly released that pressure which produced in one location a painful response. You called that finding "rebound tenderness" in the LR.

Condition	Quadrant
Acute **Pancreatitis**	UL, UR
Cholangitis	UR
Peptic **Ulcer** Disease	UL
Cholecystitis	UR
Food Poisoning	UL, UR, LR
Gastric Cancer	UL
Pancreatic Cancer	UL, UR
Hepatoma	UR
Appendicitis	LR
Intestinal **Ischemia**	UL, UR, LR
Abdominal Aortic **Aneurysm**	MIDLINE
Chronic Pancreatitis	UL, UR

The color and texture of our stools (poop) change with diet and health. Changes in a patient's stools might lead you to consider some diagnoses more likely than others:

Medical Investigation 101

Condition	Stool appearance/symptom
Acute Pancreatitis	constipation
Cholangitis	constipation
Peptic Ulcer Disease	Red, maroon, black color
Cholecystitis	constipation
Food Poisoning	diarrhea
Gastric Cancer	constipation or diarrhea
Pancreatic Cancer	oily, smelly, pale, yellow
Hepatoma	White, clay-like
Appendicitis	constipation or diarrhea
Intestinal Ischemia	constipation or diarrhea
Abdominal Aortic Aneurysm	normal
Chronic Pancreatitis	Oily, smelly, pale, yellow

We need to better understand our differential diagnostic list before moving forward with tests. Remember, the final diagnosis often results from ruling out diseases from the differential diagnosis list until only a few remain.

Acute Pancreatitis involves inflammation of the pancreas of recent onset. The pancreas manufactures digestive enzymes and insulin. Insulin controls the absorption of sugar into the cells throughout our body. Malfunction of the pancreas that reduces insulin production causes one form of the disease we call diabetes.

Cholangitis is an inflammation of the bile duct system. Usually a bacterial infection causes cholangitis. The infection may occur suddenly and then either resolve or become chronic. The bile duct system carries bile from the liver and gallbladder to the duodenum of the small intestine. Bile has the ability to dissolve the fat in our food and thus allow our stomach to digest and absorb the fat.

Peptic Ulcer Disease refers to painful sores or ulcers in the lining of the stomach or first part of the small intestine. Many factors appear to play a role in producing peptic ulcers such as excess stomach acid production from tumors, excessive use of alcohol or tobacco, or exposure to radiation, but we now know the ulceration comes about from the action of a specific bacteria, **Helicobacter pylori.**

Cholecystitis is an inflammation of the gallbladder. Your gallbladder is a small, pear-shaped organ on the right side of your abdomen tucked beneath the liver. It stores a digestive fluid made by the liver called bile and releases that bile into your small intestine when you need it for digestion of fat. Gallstones are the most common cause of cholecystitis. Why gallstones form remains a mystery. The most common sign that your patient has acute cholecystitis is abdominal pain that lasts for several hours, although gallbladder problems can produce confusing arrays of symptoms.

Food Poisoning is illness caused by ingestion of bacteria or toxins in food; typical symptoms are nausea and vomiting. As you will see when you read the chapter on food-borne illness, the duration of illness depends on which organism your patient ingests.

Gastric Cancer, growth of a tumor in the lining of the stomach, constitutes the third most common cause of cancer death in the world. Symptoms begin as indigestion and eventually become chronic stomach pain.

Pancreatic Cancer, malignant cells growing in the pancreas, underneath the stomach, commonly spreads (**metastasizes**) before it produces recognizable symptoms, leaving a rather poor prognosis for your patient by the time of diagnosis.

Hepatoma, the most common form of cancer to grow in the liver, produces few symptoms and often is diagnosed during a physical exam when palpation reveals an enlarged liver. The long-term prognosis is poor, with death often resulting in as little as one year.

Appendicitis occurs when the appendix becomes inflamed, swollen, and filled with **purulence** (commonly called pus). The appendix is a small finger-shaped structure located on the right side of the abdomen attached internally to the first portion of the colon. The exact function of the appendix remains unknown. Why it suddenly becomes infected also remains unknown. Surgeons consider appendicitis an emergency because if not removed it can rupture, spreading a life-threatening infection throughout the abdominal cavity. Symptoms of appendicitis include lower right abdominal pain, nausea, vomiting, decreased appetite, and rebound tenderness (pressure applied slowly to the abdomen then suddenly released to produce pain). Appendicitis most commonly occurs in patients between ten and thirty years of age, again for reasons that remain unknown.

Intestinal Ischemia, an inadequate blood supply to the small or large intestines caused by a blood clot or mechanical obstruction of blood flow, causes severe unrelenting abdominal pain. Severe pain can occur within minutes, often after eating, and usually in patients over age sixty.

Abdominal Aortic Aneurysm (AAA) presents as a bulging enlargement of the largest blood vessel in your body. Subtle signs such as rapid heart rate, dizziness, and sweating can occur; however, most abdominal aortic aneurysms are asymptomatic until they leak or completely rupture. You should suspect a possible AAA in your patient if you hear a rushing sound of blood (**bruit**) when listening carefully with your stethoscope over the central abdomen. Sometimes an examiner can feel an aneurysm by applying pressure over the central abdomen. An abdominal ultrasound can confirm an AAA. You don't want to miss this diagnosis. If the aneurysm ruptures your patient can die too quickly for any treatment to occur. Surgeons and radiologists can now repair many AAA's by introducing collapsed **stents** into arteries in the leg and then expanding them in the aorta.

Chronic Pancreatitis represents long-standing inflammation of the pancreas that does not improve or resolve. Long-term alcohol abuse often appears to play a role in causing this condition. Over time pancreatitis impairs the patient's ability to digest food or produce insulin. Symptoms include abdominal pain, digestive problems, and diabetes.

Even though chronic diseases begin as acute, you probably still want to rule out acute illnesses first since those conditions benefit from prompt action. **With that in mind, make a list on a piece of paper of potential causes you are willing to eliminate from your immediate evaluation plan.**

Based on what you know now, before conducting any tests, write down your top three suspects as the cause of Crystal's distress.

Medical Tests:

You have available a myriad of medical tests for gaining additional information in this investigation. You have to consider not only the amount of information gained, but also the expense and risk to the patient of each test. For example, any test utilizing x-rays requires radiation exposure that carries some risk. You must decide whether the potential information is worth the exposure the patient endures. Some of the tests you might consider for this patient are listed below.

Complete Blood Test (CBC): An elevated white cell count demonstrates infection. The CBC requires drawing blood from the patient.

CT Scan of abdomen: Utilizes high doses of radiation to provide a layer-by-layer visualization of the structures of the abdomen. Soft tissue resolution may prove lower than MRI. Your patient receives a relatively high radiation exposure.

Urinalysis: Test can be helpful in ruling out a urinary tract infection. Test looks for blood or bacteria in the urine. Patient pees into a container.

Ultrasound of abdomen: Sound waves are bounced off the abdominal structures, sending back a picture of the abdomen. Sound waves pose no risk to the patient.

X-ray of abdomen: X-rays shot through the abdomen provide a contrasting view of boney versus soft tissue structures in the abdomen. Definition of soft tissue abnormality may prove limited. Patient is exposed to x-rays.

MRI of abdomen: An MRI uses a strong magnetic field to create high resolution images of soft tissue structures. It is safer than X-rays, but much more expensive than x-rays or ultrasound. MRI cannot be used freely in patients with cardiac pacemakers or metal implants.

Think about and list on a piece of paper the medical test or tests you would order for this patient.

Medical Investigation 101

Note: Emergency physicians increasingly use CT scans and sometimes MRI scans to sort out difficult cases of suspected appendicitis. These modalities have a higher accuracy rate than other imaging methods, so you may have a family member who underwent one of these studies to sort out acute abdominal discomfort.

Review of History: Let's do a quick review of Crystal's history as stated by her Mother.

1. Very recent onset
2. No friends had same symptoms
3. Pain lower right quadrant of abdomen, radiating to right side
4. Nausea & sweating
5. Bloating
6. Increased pain on moving

Review of Examination findings: Here is a summary of the exam findings.

1. Temperature 101.9
2. Pulse 92 bpm
3. Respirations 22 / min
4. Yellowish color to eye sclera
5. Absent bowel sounds
6. Rebound tenderness

Medical Test Results

If you ordered a CBC: elevated white cell count   Note... a sed rate is not commonly part of a CBC

If you ordered a Urinalysis: no blood or bacteria found in the urine.

If you ordered an Ultrasound of the Abdomen: **dilated** appendix with **peri-appendiceal** fluid. The wall layers of the appendix are visible. Remaining abdominal structures are within normal limits.

Based on your examination findings and laboratory tests, what is your Preliminary Diagnosis?

Treatment

Treatment of appendicitis usually results in surgical removal of the appendix, a relatively minor operation, with the goal of preventing rupture and spread of infection. Patients with mild symptoms and no confirming studies may receive antibiotics, and if symptoms continue or worsen undergo an **appendectomy**.

Any surgery has inherent risks for which your attending surgeon must be vigilant. Fortunately, appendectomy enjoys a relatively low frequency of complications. However, a ruptured appendix possesses a severe threat to life. Treating appendicitis with antibiotics alone has a 58.3% success rate, meaning about 42% of those patients end up having surgery, with a 92.6% success for those patients. A clear diagnosis of appendicitis in an otherwise healthy patient should result in a quick trip to an operating room. Have any of your friends had their appendix removed?

Investigation 3.2B: Microbes

English teachers often introduce students to journalistic writing by suggesting that the author must explain to the reader "who, what, when, where, why, and how." Which of those elements would you rate the most complex or difficult to explain? *How* can sometimes prove a challenge, but most authors seem to work the hardest to figure out *why*. Human beings appear unique in the ranks of living organisms in their endless quest to puzzle over *why*. Why is the sky blue? *Why* does the letter Q always need a U? Why does ice float?

We apparently were born with an instinct for asking *why*. A biologist might argue that asking *why* created an **evolutionary** advantage for the human species. We have certainly begun to see that asking *why* plays a huge role in medical science. Let's follow the role of human curiosity in regard to microbes. Let's turn the clock back 500 years and consider what *"why"* questions you might then have asked. Life is very different for you 500 years ago. No one yells at you to brush your teeth. That habit did not exist. Lacking automobiles, you did not travel long distances easily. Back then you would notice that people, young and old, commonly got sick and quite commonly died from any significant illness. Doctors and nurses existed, but they believed disease came from **miasma**. Miasma? Curious people back then noticed that illness seemed associated with impurity, poor cleanliness, or foul-smelling air. Thus, they concluded that foul air caused illness. They called the origin of disease miasma, an ancient Greek word meaning foul or bad air.

Pretend your teacher back then believed in homework and assigned you the task of figuring out *why* some stale bread made everyone who ate it sick, but no one who ate the fresh bread two days before got sick. How might you attack that homework assignment?

Teachers sometimes give you a choice for special homework projects. Alternatively, you might have been asked to figure out *how* two people many miles apart could come down with the same set of disease symptoms, people who never met each other or shared any contact with the same miasma. How might you start to figure out that puzzle?

Amazingly 68-year-old, Girolamo **Fracastoro**, an Italian scholar assigned himself that very same homework assignment. He decided miasma made no sense at all. In 1546, he instead suggested that some sort of invisible seed must transmit illnesses. How could he prove that something invisible actually existed? What would lead him to even conjecture the existence of something solid, like a seed, with the ability to make people sick, yet the eye could not see it? Fracastoro had an unusual imagination.

Today we generally think of Louis **Pasteur** as the scientist first to understand the real origin of infectious disease. Pasteur performed experiments that linked germs to human illness, but Pasteur did that in about 1860, more than three hundred years after the period you just time traveled into. Pasteur, by then, had the benefit of Anton van Leeuwenhoek's invention. About 1670, **Leeuwenhoek** figured out how to use magnifying glasses to see tiny living things, **microorganisms**, never actually seen by anyone before. Leeuwenhoek saw germs 190 years before Pasteur linked them to disease. Leeuwenhoek made microbes visible; so why did it take 190 years to make the connection between microbes and illness? Actually, other scientists did put pieces of the puzzle together much earlier; but science still seems to have moved more slowly than we might imagine, perhaps because methods for rapidly sharing ideas and discoveries we take for granted today, did not exist then.

The years between 1860 and 1900 saw the growth of human knowledge of **germs** as a cause of disease. Robert **Koch** became a star in this area of knowledge by creating a set of rules one could use to prove a specific germ caused a specific disease by analyzing sets of specific symptoms. The rules were pretty straight forward:

Rule 1: A person with the disease must have lots of this germ, but healthy people have none.

Rule 2: You must be able to isolate the germ and grow it in a germ culture in your laboratory.

Rule 3: If you give those cultured germs to a healthy person they must get the same disease.

Rule 4: You must be able to get germs back from the person you made sick, grow them in culture, and see that they look the same as the germs you cultured back in Rule 2.

Do Koch's rules remain true for us today? They seem to make sense, but today we recognize some exceptions. Can you think of an exception?

Koch's Rule 1 failed for him fairly early after he created them because **cholera** and typhoid fever, Koch discovered, had carriers. A **carrier** we define as a person who does not have the symptoms of the disease but can spread the disease to others. Mary Mallon's bizarre story took place in New York City in the first decade of the 20th century. Mary Mallon, known as **Typhoid Mary**, spread the deadly disease **typhoid fever** but did not have the disease herself. She was imprisoned for many years to stop her from spreading the disease and the story of her life seems impossible for us to comprehend today.

We also recognize now that some people can resist a disease that makes others sick, so Rule 3 has exceptions. We know that some people can have **immunity** to a disease that others do not; indeed, we know that vaccination can create immunity to a disease.

The second half of the 19th century (1850 – 1899) saw the rapid growth of human knowledge about germs as a cause of disease and using a **microscope,** scientists could see those germs and could see them grow and divide to form increasing numbers of identical germs in a culture dish in the laboratory. These scientists understood that germs were alive, consisted of a single cell, and they used food to create energy for a biochemical process of growth similar to the functioning of cells in our own bodies.

As these scientists kept asking why, new questions arose. Near the end of the 19th century a French microbiologist invented a **membrane** with **pores** that could allow a fluid to pass through, but the pores were too small for a germ to cross. About the same time, Louis Pasteur failed to find a germ that caused **rabies;** he began to think something smaller than a germ must exist to cause that disease. Several other scientists around the world started to find diseases that were caused by something that could pass through the pores in that membrane. By 1928, the concept of a **virus,** something smaller than a germ but able to induce a disease, was widely accepted, but still no one had seen a virus. Not until 1931, with the German invention of the **electron microscope**, did humans have the ability to "see" a virus and begin to understand this simpler, smaller structure able to cause illness. In the 1970's scientists began to understand the chemistry by which viruses translate their genes into the genes of host cells that then create more viruses. We now had an understanding of how both viruses and bacteria survive and cause disease.

Bacteria, fungi and viruses, along with several less common single cell organisms, all individually too small for us to see, biologists group together in a category they call **microbes**. Microbes live all around us on the ground, in the ground, in the air, on us, and inside us. Biologists have estimated that we have more microbes on our skin than the total population of people living on this planet. We need microbes to live, but microbes do not appear to need humans. Microbes, we believe, began living on earth long, long before human life. Let's take a look at some of the similarities and differences between two principle types of microbes, bacteria and viruses.

First, biologists have found that a virus does not exhibit all the behaviors we call "life." Bacteria, on the other hand, do exhibit life, having everything necessary to live and grow with or without the help of another living host (another living organism). For example, we can stick a sterile Q-tip into an infected area on an animal or human and send that sample to a medical laboratory, where technicians can actually grow more of the bacteria in a dish containing only some simple germ friendly food. Laboratory technicians can then identify exactly which bacteria infected that wound. They cannot grow a virus in that manner. A virus needs more than just food to grow. Viruses are not considered living things because they cannot reproduce, and thus survive, without a living host (like us). Viruses reproduce by invading living cells and using the capabilities of those cells to manufacture similar viruses, until the cell dies.

When asked about your size, you might tell someone your height in feet and inches. In the world of microbes, scientists measure things in **nanometers** (a billion nanometers equal one meter in length). Put another way, 25 million 400 thousand nanometers equal one inch. A typical bacterium (the singular form of the word bacteria) measures about 1,000 nanometers. If you lined up bacteria in single file you would need 25,400 to make the line one inch long, or about 645 million bacteria to cover a one-inch square area. Now if we could shrink you down to the size of a typical bacterium, and put you next to a typical virus, that virus would look to you about the size of a small mouse. The unaided human eye cannot see objects less than 40,000 nanometers readily, so you certainly cannot see individual microbes. You can see a bacterium with an optical microscope, but not a virus.

Bacteria, you now recognize, have much greater complexity than viruses. Bacteria have a rigid cell wall and cytoplasm inside containing mitochondria and DNA. Viruses have only a protein coat, either RNA or DNA inside, and nothing else.

We tend to think of bacteria only as the cause of harmful infection. But in truth, most bacteria prove helpful; indeed, human beings cannot live without the help of bacteria. Only about 1% of bacteria actually cause human disease. Scientists currently believe most viruses do cause harm. However, as we look into the future of medical research, we may see viruses helping cure sickness, disease, and even genetic disorders. As you will read later in this book, finding helpful roles for viruses has already begun. We can create a virus in the laboratory that can invade cells to correct defective genes. Scientists have begun to understand that a virus can store useful traits that can help living cells adapt to changes in their environment. Some viruses in the plant world transmit the ability for plants to withstand severe drought, for example. It would appear that such viruses play the role of an outsourced set of plant skills, ready when needed to infect and assist the plant. We may in the future find that viruses play similarly useful, even necessary roles, in human life in this same fashion. The role that helpful viruses may play in our lives remains a compelling topic for medical research in the future.

Bacteria and viruses have been around for billions of years; they occur wherever life exists. They have caused an inordinate amount of sickness and death throughout the centuries. Both continue to survive due to their extraordinary ability to adapt to their changing environment. Their amazing ability to adapt and evolve results from their very rapid reproductive cycle, as compared to the much longer reproductive cycle of complex animals, including humans. Even when we think a harmful bacteria or virus has been eradicated, they seem to re-emerge, sometimes years later.

In 1928, Alexander Fleming discovered a mold that killed bacteria growing near it in a dish used to grow microbes in his laboratory. That mold produced a juice that Fleming named **Penicillin**. Penicillin, the first ever **antibiotic,** signaled an historic advance in medical treatment. Scientists went on to develop many other antibiotic medications that controlled most bacterial infections for years. Today we find that antibiotics have been overused, and bacteria have evolved antibiotic resistance so that many of our antibiotics no longer work. Indeed we now have strains of bacteria causing **super-infections** resistant to all antibiotics. We have essentially returned to the situation humans faced before Fleming discovered Penicillin. We hope that scientists can quickly develop yet newer antibiotics effective against these super-infections. So please don't ask your doctor for antibiotics every time you catch a cold. Antibiotics do not help you overcome an illness caused by a virus. We do now have anti-viral medicines available that may help if taken in the first day or two of a viral infection. Our fight against viral infections generally focuses on prevention with a **vaccine**. Once contracted, we commonly direct treatment of a viral illness to relieving the symptoms until the illness runs its course.

Medical Investigation 101

We say that bacteria and viruses both are **communicable**, meaning they can spread from one human to another. Methods of spreading an illness include breathing in microbes, touching contaminated objects, animal or bug bites, or eating contaminated food or water. Bacteria and viruses may cause sickness that is mild, moderate, severe, or even fatal. All you need to do to prevent getting sick is 1. Stop breathing, 2. Don't touch anything, 3. Don't eat food or drink water, and 4. Don't go outside. Good luck with that approach.

Let's introduce you to some infectious diseases caused by microbes.

The common cold is an airborne, mild illness caused by a virus. The **flu**, a different airborne virus, also causes a mild to fatal **febrile** illness. Probably more people have died worldwide in the past 100 years from the flu than any other disease. More soldiers died from the 1918 flu **pandemic** during World War I, than died in combat.

Chicken pox is an airborne virus common in children, but which can also infect adults. The virus can remain dormant in the body for decades and may reappear as Shingles, a painful skin condition.

Insects, such as mosquitos, spread some very serious viral infections. Dengue Fever, Yellow Fever, West Nile, and more recently Zika virus, all are spread by mosquito bites. **Zika** is thought to cause a serious problem for pregnant women by affecting the developing fetus to produce a deformity called microcephaly. A student of one of the authors contracted encephalitis caused by the West Nile virus, and missed the entire school year. Unfortunately, that student has not fully recovered and his life has been forever changed from a single mosquito bite.

Animals can spread viral diseases to humans. **Rabies** was made famous many years ago in the movie *Old Yeller*; a boy's dog contracted rabies fighting a rabid wolf while protecting his master. Old Yeller had to be put down when he started foaming at the mouth and acting crazy. Rabies can only survive in mammals, most commonly in skunks, raccoons, bats, foxes, and coyotes according to the CDC. You can't get rabies from birds, fish, or amphibians. When a person is bitten or scratched by an animal suspected of rabies, **preventive** treatment consisting of five shots given over twenty-eight days plus rabies antibodies are given. Once the signs and symptoms of rabies appear, there is no treatment; death is usually the result.

Hepatitis is a human-to-human viral infection that seeks out the liver. Several strains of hepatitis have evolved. In 2014 a new virus was discovered and named the Bourbon Virus after the county in Kansas where the infected man lived. You can look it up: Bourbon County, Kansas, USA.

Two more viruses having lethal abilities are **HIV** and **Ebola**. Both viruses are thought to have moved from the animal world of Africa to humans and then spread by human-to-human contact of bodily fluids.

Bacteria have more methods than viruses by which to spread because they can survive independently of human, mosquito or tick hosts. Ticks carry bacterium causing Lyme Disease and Rocky Mountain Spotted Fever, each common in specific areas of the United States. We can also contract bacterial diseases from food and water, even though food and water are not living carriers of infection.

How do we contract dangerous bacterial infections from our food or water? Remember microbes cover our planet. Bacteria occur naturally in the soil, and furthermore, in and on our body. When we process food without thorough cleaning, bacteria may not only survive, but also can multiply and grow. Then when we eat that food we ingest the bacteria. If that bacterium has the ability to cause illness, human beings may become ill and sometimes die.

We cannot live without water; yet contaminated water kills over a million people each year around the world. Water generally becomes contaminated in places where human and animal feces leak into the water. Organisms such as the cholera bacteria flourish in this instance. Cholera produces severe diarrhea, and massive loss of water from the colon can lead to death. The **Protozoans,** Amoebiasis and Giardiasis, single-celled organisms that biologists classify as neither a bacterium nor a virus, can also cause water-borne illness. You may have read about the rare occurrence of children getting sick and dying after swimming in warm-water lakes. Amoebas have the ability to penetrate the brain when present in water that splashes up into our noses. These children died because the organism infected their brains. **Epidemiologists** report that another protozoan causes **Malaria** and spreads the disease by mosquitoes, killing more than 1,000 children per day around the world.

Viruses, such as **polio** and **hepatitis**, also have the ability to spread in water. In the 1950's, polio spread in public swimming pools. Thousands of children contracted the disease. Those developing the most severe symptoms suffered respiratory paralysis and required the help of an iron lung to breathe. Many polio victims suffered lifelong disabilities; boys were affected with **unilateral** muscle wasting and **paralysis** while girls were left with severe **scoliosis**. Following the development of an effective **vaccine**, polio was essentially wiped out. The success of the vaccine resulted in discontinued universal use of the polio vaccine; sadly, polio has since re-emerged as a **viable** disease. Although the reason remains unclear, polio patients can experience progressive muscle weakness and atrophy, even difficulty breathing and swallowing years later, a so-called post-polio **syndrome**.

Eating contaminated food can poison our bodies, an event we call a foodborne pathogen outbreak. A foodborne outbreak occurs when two or more people get the same illness from the same food. Several types of bacteria have been proven responsible for foodborne outbreaks, but the two most prolific ones are E.Coli and Salmonella. E.Coli, short for Enterobacter Coli, has been at the root of several major food poisoning events at restaurants across our country and throughout the world. Surprisingly, E.Coli can live quite normally within our body, and yet has also made millions sick, even causing death over the years.

We have talked about the airborne spread of infections. Bacteria can invade our body when exhaled by a sick person and breathed in as we innocently walk by. **Tuberculosis** is a serious lung infection spread when infected individuals cough. This disease, often called simply TB, was at one time so difficult to treat that those infected where isolated, sometimes against their will, in special hospitals. Today we have a vaccine that can prevent TB, but experts recommend the use of this vaccine only in areas of the world with very high TB prevalence.

We can infect ourselves also directly by touching things recently touched by another infected person. Staphylococcus and Streptococcus are bacteria that spread in that way. Staphylococcus causes **abscesses** when we don't properly clean a cut or scratch, or when it infects our tonsils. Streptococcus can spread from a wound or cause "strep throat".

In summary, we have learned that microbes, whether living single cell organisms or just packets of genetic material not truly alive, surround us and can cause illness. We also know that humans require microbes to survive; we need them to digest our food and to do other tasks inside our bodies, functions still emerging today from medical research. Plants and animals that humans need for food also depend on microbes. Microbes in the roots of pea plants carry out chemical reactions that give that vegetable its nutrient value. Plants may depend on traits encoded in viruses to help them survive a drought. In the future we will probably discover humans also benefit from viral interactions. Medical scientists have begun to use laboratory-engineered viruses as a way to edit genes in plants, animals, and humans to enhance illness resistance, increase food production, restrict disease spread, and correct congenital defects. Today microbiologists estimate that the mass of the microbes within the earth's crust actually exceed the mass of living organisms on the earth's surface. We have great concerns about global warming that initially focused entirely on energy use, but now our concerns have centered on the effects on microbial population shifts that may have even more crucial impact on human life. We need to understand that humans, animals, plants, and microbes live in equilibrium and synergy with each other and those relationships contain both promise and danger. Indeed, of those four components of our world, the microbes would appear to have the least dependency on the other three. We all need to continue to ask *"why."*

Medical Investigation 101

[For a complete list of communicable diseases please consult the CDC, the Communicable Disease Center of our federal government at www.cdc.gov. This is an excellent place to learn about microbes and about recent epidemics of food-borne pathogens.]

Investigation 3.3

3.3A: Rib Area Pain

3.3B: Shingles

Investigation 3.3A: Rib Area Pain

Introduction:

When a patient presents with pain in their chest or ribs, as their physician, you must sort out the origin of that pain. Does their pain come from the skin overlying the ribs, from the muscles between the ribs, from the organs directly under the ribs, or from the ribs themselves?

The ribs function as a protective boney cage that guards the vital organs beneath. If you get hit in the ribs by a ninety-mile-per-hour fastball, the impact can break one or more ribs and injure the organs below. If the rib breaks completely it can puncture a lung, a very serious injury. Sometimes a rib can **fracture** simply from turning in such a way as to put too much stress on the weakest part of this long, thin, curved bone. But many other conditions can cause pain in the area of the ribs. Your job, as always, is to investigate the possibilities and come up with the diagnosis.

You have enjoyed a wonderful few days off, but today you must head to the office and pay the price. Whenever you take a holiday the first day back in the office proves exhausting, because you need to see everyone in your practice who has developed new symptoms while you relaxed. As you come through the door your medical office receptionist shoves the list of appointments at you before even saying, "Welcome back." You understand, of course, that your receptionist has spent hours on the telephone with your patients trying to make sure everyone with urgent needs got the attention of the doctor who routinely covers for you. If the symptoms did not seem urgent, that patient went on your list.

The first name on the list actually pleases you. Professor Edwin Bristol, retired, a computer scientist, makes you glad to have your job because he always gives you a thorough history and sincerely appreciates your efforts to keep him healthy and active.

Chief Complaint:

Today Ed sits on the examination table in Exam Room 1 and is not displaying his characteristic smile and jovial nature. "What's wrong Ed?" you ask.

He answers, "Doc, I have been in misery for two days. I have a burning pain in my ribs on the right side that will not go away. I can't sleep. I have no **appetite**. All I can do is sit in my chair and suffer."

You quickly review the new chart notes left by your nurse:

Weight: 178   BP: 158/92   Pulse: 88   Respirations: 19   Temp: 98.4 F.

Then you ask, "What started this Ed?"

"I don't know. I don't remember anything hitting my ribs. I did move some furniture for my wife about four days ago, but I don't remember feeling like anything strained or pulled while I was helping her. I can't figure it out."

You are thinking very hard about what could be happening to Ed.

What Ed says next explains why Ed has become a favorite patient of yours. He uses his computer skills to try to figure out himself what has happened to his body.

"I ran my symptoms through the Isabel Healthcare symptom checker on the internet *[http://symptomchecker.isabelhealthcare.com/home/products]* and they said I might have **fibromyalgia**, food poisoning, vitamin B12 deficiency, lung cancer, **depression**, restless leg **syndrome**, a **brachial plexus** injury, **concussion**, mono-**neuropathy** multiplex, sleep **apnea**, **shingles**, **stroke**, **multiple sclerosis**, general **anxiety** disorder, iron deficiency **anemia**, or about 20 other things that included diabetic neuropathy. I do have that borderline Type II **Diabetes** that you found, but I am staying on the diet you gave me. Could this be coming from my diabetes?"

The Isabel Healthcare website had certainly kicked out a wide array of possible causes for Ed's chief complaint. You know your knowledge and diagnostic skills will be tested to whittle down that list into a workable differential diagnosis in order to come up with the diagnosis and treatment.

You next get Ed to remove his shirt. After a quick exam of his normal heart and lungs you ask him to point out where he feels his discomfort. There is not much to see. Ed has dark skin and it looks perfectly normal. You **palpate** along the right T-6 rib and Ed confirms you got the right area, but your touch does not seem to **elicit** worse pain. The area of discomfort seems to follow along that single rib perhaps 6-8 inches in length. Nothing appears bruised or injured anywhere else on his arms or **thorax**. Lymph nodes in the right armpit are not **palpable** or enlarged.

You clearly want to figure out the cause so you can get Ed back to normal, but you do not see anything life threatening, and this day in the office has a full schedule. So, you decide to give Ed some serious pain medicine so he can sleep and ask him to come back to see you in two days. You tell Ed that a strained muscle or a sprain will resolve and the pain medicine will allow time for that to happen. If the pain persists you will need to do a more thorough examination and some extensive testing, but it will take time to set all of that up. In the meantime, you ask him to call the office if anything changes.

The rest of the day meets your expectations of hectic. You drag yourself home at its end, and head to bed much earlier than usual. The next morning when you sit down at your desk to start another day at your office, you see a note from your receptionist that says Ed's wife phoned to say Ed has a rash and a few blisters all along that rib, and it still hurts. He experienced diarrhea this morning as well. Are these new clues helpful in making your diagnosis?

Review of Systems:

A review of Ed's medical history reveals that he had measles and chicken pox as a child. Your chart indicates he is borderline diabetic and he has managed his diabetes as your patient of the past 9 years with strict diet control. He has no history of fractured ribs, abdominal pain, or chest pain.

Examination:

Wt: 178 lbs.   Respirations: 19 /min   Pulse: 88 /min
Blood Pressure: 158/92   Temperature: 98.5° F.

Heart: no abnormal sounds

Lungs: clear

Chest exam:

- pain elicited on palpation along the right T-6 rib for a distance of 6 – 8 inches.
- No sign of bruising or other discoloration.
- No enlarged lymph nodes right armpit. Lymph nodes for the area of Ed's pain lie inside the chest and thus one cannot examine them directly.
- No palpable mass

Remainder of exam deferred until next visit.

Differential Diagnosis: The following chart contains some of the possible conditions that may cause similar symptoms.

U = unilateral   B = bilateral

Disorder	Acute/ Chronic	Pain ↑ moving/ breathing	Swollen lymph nodes	Head aches	rash	Uni or bi-lateral	Stiff joints	Numb ness	blisters	Dia-rhea
Muscle strain	A	X				U				
Rib Fracture	A	X				U		X		
Fibromyalgia	C	X		X		U/B	X			X
Food poisoning	A		X	X						X
Lung Cancer	C	X	X							
Brachial plexus injury	A	X				U		X		
Shingles	A/C		X		X	U		X	X	X
Stroke	A/C					U		X		
Multiple sclerosis	C	X				U/B				

Medical Investigation 101

Medical Tests: Below are some of the medical tests you might consider to assist in your investigation.

Complete Blood Count (CBC)	High WBC count suggests infection; Low WBC count suggests immune response suppression
Biopsy of rib	A sample of rib bone is taken and examined for signs of cancer or other abnormality
Magnetic Resonance Imaging (MRI) of chest/ribs	Provides a layer by layer view of the entire chest area to visualize an intercostal cartilage tear or other soft tissue abnormality
Prescription for pain medication	Blocks pain but does not cure the problem
Ultrasound of chest/ribs	Uses sound to visualize the soft tissue structures of the chest
X-Ray of ribs	Shows boney structures to rule out fracture
CT Scan of ribs	Uses high doses of radiation to detect rib fractures not seen on x-ray or enlarged lymph nodes.

Which test(s) would be most appropriate at this time? (Copy the following list and circle those you would consider ordering for this patient.)

- **X-rays** of the chest and ribs
- **MRI** of the chest and ribs
- **Rib Biopsy**
- **CBC** blood test
- **Ultrasound** of chest and ribs
- **Prescription** for pain medication

Test Results:

If you ordered a chest x-ray your report would read something like this: No fractures of dislocations are visualized. The pleural cavities are clear. Normal chest x-ray.

Diagnosis:

Ed is counting on you to make the diagnosis! Was there a particular clue that really brought this investigation into focus for you? What is your diagnosis? As it turns out, none of the tests available to you would have provided the diagnosis. Sometimes information obtained from the patient is your best investigative tool.

Investigation 3.3B: Shingles

Have you had **Chicken Pox**? Hopefully not, since there is a **vaccination** that can prevent you ever contracting this viral disease. Ask your parents if you have been vaccinated. But what about your parents and grandparents? When your grandparents were growing up no vaccine existed to prevent chicken pox. If your grandparents had chicken pox, then they are **susceptible** to Shingles.

The **varicella-zoster** virus causes chicken pox. This virus continues to reside in your body even after you fight off the illness. Varicella-zoster can remain **dormant** for years upon years. About **one-third** of chicken pox victims develop Shingles many years later. In fact, most patients suffering from Shingles are over 60 years old. It is rare to see a patient with Shingles under the age of 40.

So how does **Shingles** occur? After many years the virus becomes active again in some people. When this happens, the patient feels pain, itching, or tingling in the area where a rash will occur in the next few days on one side of the body or face. After the rash appears, within a few days blisters can form at the rash site. The patient might also have a slight fever, headaches, chills, or an upset stomach. The **blisters** scab over in seven to ten days and go away in two to four weeks. During this time the area can remain very painful - indeed the pain can last long after the scabs resolve. When the pain lasts after the **rash** has disappeared it is called post-herpetic **neuralgia** (PHN). Very rarely Shingles can progress to cause **blindness**, hearing loss, **pneumonia**, or **encephalitis**, even death.

The good news is that Shingles is now **preventable**; your parents and grandparents don't have to be victims of Shingles. The Shingles **vaccine** prevents the virus from re-activating. But waiting until Shingles occurs does not work; the **vaccination** must be given before Shingles occurs.

Shingles cannot be passed on to others; but the varicella virus causing chickenpox can. Shingles blisters contain the virus, so it is important to prevent the spread of chickenpox by covering the rash and blisters of Shingles. Pregnant women and people with weak **immune systems**, such as cancer patients, patients taking **steroid** medications, and organ **transplant** patients are at higher risk of contracting chickenpox from contact with the virus in the blisters if they have not yet had it. However, in general, Shingles is less contagious than chickenpox. Don't let your grandparents get Shingles; ask them to get vaccinated!

Investigation 3.4

3.4A: Sore Throat

3.4B: Role of Blood

Investigation 3.4A: Sore Throat

Introduction:

Sore throats cause almost a quarter million patient visits to their doctors each year. Even doctors come down with a sore throat from time to time. A sore throat is often the first sign of a cold. A virus causes most sore throats and they last about ten days with or without supportive care (bed rest, salt water gargles, antihistamines, cough syrup, and anti-inflammatory medicines. But other illnesses also cause sore throats; so, if your patient has a temperature of 101 F. or higher, you need to see them.

Chief Complaint:

Ronald, a thirteen-year-old boy, is brought to see you by his Mother. Ronald has a sore throat that started four days ago. Ronald reports the right side of his throat hurts more than the left side. He complains of losing his voice, smelling his own bad breath, and not feeling hungry. He also reports experiencing headaches and alternating feelings of chills and fever.

His Mother tells you that he has experienced similar throat infections at least nine times over the past three years. As a result, he has missed many days of school, which has caused Ronald great concern because it affected his grades. Mom also states this is the third time this year Ronald has had a similar infection. Mom further reports that Ronald snores loudly only when he has throat infections. Ronald had a physician caring for this condition, but they have moved recently and would like you to take over his care. Ronald enjoys playing soccer and playing video games. He makes good grades in school except when he doesn't feel well from his throat infections.

Review of Systems:

Ronald's Mother again says that Ronald has had at least nine throat infections over the past three years. Ronald occasionally has a nosebleed, especially in warm weather months. His Mother denies any episodes of uncontrollable bleeding. Ronald has no surgical history. Ronald has experienced an allergic reaction to sulfa-based antibiotics but has no other known allergies.

Examination:

Ht = 66 in.   Wt = 140 lbs.   Respirations: 18/min   Pulse: 76
Blood Pressure is 98/60. Temperature = 102.4° F.

Head and Neck:

Eyes: erythema and **glassy** appearance

Ears: erythema of **tympanic membrane**

Mouth: Enlargement of both **tonsils** and **erythema** of the tonsillar bed and surrounding tissues. A small amount of yellowish **purulent discharge** with an **abscess** is noted on the right **tonsil**. Teeth are aligned normally. The **Uvula** appears swollen and erythematous.

Neck: Enlargement of **lymph nodes** on both sides of the neck

Heart: Heart sounds normal

Lungs: Breath sounds normal all quadrants

Abdomen: Bowel sounds active.

Extremities: Normal appearance. **Reflexes** and **pulses** within normal limits.

Differential Diagnosis:

	Acute/ chronic	Sore throat	Fever	Enlarged Tonsils	Enlarged lymph nodes	Purulent Discharge	Ear Ache	Pos. C&S	Fatigue	Rash Neck & Chest
Bacterial Tonsillitis	A	x	x	x	x	x	x	x	x	
Strept Throat	A	x	x		x			x	x	
Mononucleosis	AC	x	x	x	x			x	x	x
Lymphoma	C		x	x	x			x	x	
Tooth Abscess	AC		x		x	x		x	x	
Carcinoma	C			x	x				x	
Diptheria	A	x	x		x	x		x	x	
Scarlet Fever	A	x	x		x			x	x	x
Viral Tonsillitis	A	x	x	x	x		x		x	

Review of medical records:

Because the patient had a physician treating this condition over the past three years, you want to examine the old records. If you confirm that Ronald has experienced Tonsillitis nine times in three years, you may want to recommend he undergo surgical removal of his tonsils. If not you would recommend a more conservative approach to solving this medical investigation. While waiting for the medical records to arrive you must treat his current condition.

Medical Tests

Look at the summary of available tests to consider how they can help your medical investigation:

Complete Blood Count (CBC)	High WBC count suggests infection; Low WBC count suggests immune response suppression
Culture & Sensitivity (C&S) of throat	Test which germs grow & which antibiotics will control them
Magnetic Resonance Imaging (MRI) of Neck	Provides a layer by layer view of the entire throat area
Prescription for Antibiotic	Kills or blocks reproduction of certain bacteria
Ultrasound of Neck	Uses sound to visualize the structures of the throat
X-Ray of Neck	Shows the boney structures of mouth & neck

Think about which test(s) would be most appropriate at this time? (write your choices on your paper)

- **X-rays** of the head and neck
- **MRI** of the head and neck
- **Culture and Sensitivity**
- **CBC** blood test
- **Ultrasound** of neck

Treatment Options:

Think about which treatment you would prescribe while waiting for test results:

- Emergency **Surgery** to remove the infected and swollen tonsil.

Medical Investigation 101

- o **Radiation therapy** to knock out whatever is causing the tonsils to enlarge.
- o **Prescription** for a broad spectrum **Antibiotic** that works on several potential causes of infection including your first choice from your differential list.
- o **Prescriptions for all antibiotics** that work on the four most common organisms causing infections.
- o **No prescriptions** until all tests come back with results on the organism

Test results:

After two days your test results come back from the lab and indicate Ronald's tonsillitis is caused by a bacterial infection of the staph aureus organism. The sensitivity report indicates the organism is **sensitive** to the antibiotic you prescribed. This means your treatment should be effective. What would you do if the C&S report indicated the antibiotic you chose was NOT effective?

When Ronald's medical records arrive from the other physician one week later you find chart notations for at least nine episodes of tonsillitis over the past three years. The American Medical Association criteria for **tonsillectomy,** surgical removal of the tonsils, is as follows:

A. 7 episodes of tonsillitis in 1 year, or
B. 5 episodes per year for consecutive 2 years, or
C. 3 episodes per year for consecutive 3 years

Treatment Options: The following chart list some of the treatments used to treat the problems listed in your differential diagnosis.

Pathology	Cause	Treatment
Strept Infection	Streptococcus bacteria	Penicillin, amoxicillin, cephalexin
Mononucleosis	Epstein-Barr virus (EBV)	Virus; no specific treatment
Lymphoma	Helicobactor Pylori	Chemotherapy, radiation
Carcinoma	Genetic mutations	Chemotherapy, radiation
Abscess	Staph aureus bacteria	Cephalexin, Nafcillin, Vancomycin
Diptheria	Corynebacterium	Antitoxin, Penicillin, Erythromycin
Scarlet Fever	Streptococcus bacteria	Penicillin, Amoxicillin, Cephalexin

Which treatment might you prescribe first? Based on Ronald's history, what else might you recommend for a long term solution for Ronald's recurring condition?

Additional food for thought:

You likely recognized that Ronald had an infection, probably suggested to you by his symptoms of fever and chills. Your body maintains its **internal** temperature remarkably constant, unlike some animals like reptiles that we call "cold blooded." But why would temperature control prove so important to humans? We mentioned briefly before that the cells in our body carry out all sorts of chemical reactions that allow us to move about, heal ourselves, remember things, think, speak, and grow. These chemical reactions that would require high temperatures if we tried to carry them out in a laboratory test tube, take place inside our bodies at a lower temperature because of the **enzymes** coded in our human genes and manufactured inside our cells. You might think of these enzymes as fingers or molds that can hold other molecules close together in a way that allows them to chemically bond or in other cases break apart to form new molecules at our body's normal temperature. These chemical reactions constitute the core of what it means to be alive. Our amazing human enzymes have evolved to work most efficiently at 98.7 degrees Fahrenheit, our normal body (core) temperature.

Germs or viruses that invade our body commonly create protein molecules called **pyrogens**. These **pyrogens** mix with our blood and travel about our body in order to disrupt our temperature control system that has its headquarters inside our brain. The control center, when disrupted, mistakenly believes our body has gotten too cold so it orders up chills and shivering to increase our internal temperature, thus we develop a fever. Similarly when we treat the fever or resolve the infection, we often experience sweating as the temperature control system gets back to working correctly and sets about to bring our body temperature back down to 98.7. You might reason that germs and viruses go to the trouble of confusing our temperature controls to gain some advantage for themselves, and physicians would agree with you. The advantages might prove varied and numerous in specific infections. Indeed, we probably do not fully understand all of them. We do believe in general that our ability to defend ourselves against **pathogenic** germs and viruses suffers when the higher temperature of a fever moves our enzymes away from their most efficient, normal zone of operation.

Notice that we used the term **pathogenic** germs and viruses. Pathogenic means the ones that harm us. You may have the impression that all germs and viruses harm us, but science is learning right now more and more about how non-pathogenic germs and viruses actually play vital roles inside our body. We now believe a healthy adult human has more than 5 pounds of germs inside them contributing to their well-being in a variety of ways that we are only beginning to fully understand. A whole new branch of medical science is emerging around the role bacteria play inside our intestines, bacteria that clearly help us digest our food, but also may regulate many other human functions even to include our mood. Watch for new information about this fascinating area of medical research in the future that is unraveling the dependence of our body on germs and viruses that help us out.

Investigation 3.4B: The Role of Blood

Now that we have used an examination of Ronald's **blood** to help us solve this investigation, let's look more deeply into what a laboratory can learn from a blood sample.

In addition to our examination findings, we asked our nurse to take a sample of blood from Ronald's arm. That blood sample was sent to a laboratory that specializes in analyzing **blood**. Technicians at the lab can look at the blood under a microscope and **estimate** the numbers of each of the types of blood cells in the specimen to gain information about how Ronald's body is reacting to his illness. Today, we also have the ability to analyze blood using computerized banks of sensors. How does that work, you ask?

By looking at the blood of thousands of 'normal' people, we have been able to learn what 'normal blood' looks like. We then **compare** 'normal' blood to the blood samples received from sick patients and see how they are different.

What types of cells are found in blood? First, there are three basic parts to blood:

1. **Plasma**
2. **White Blood Cells** & **Platelets**
3. **Red Blood Cells**

Each of the parts has a basic responsibility in our bodies. Blood can be separated into the three basic parts by spinning the samples in a **centrifuge**. Why do you think the blood parts separate by the process of spinning?

Look at the blood specimen in the tube below. Notice there are three separate layers after blood is spun in a centrifuge.

Medical Investigation 101

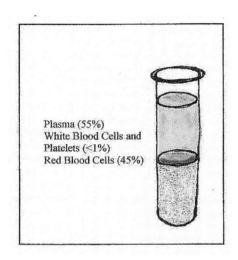

So, what is the job of each?

Let's start with **plasma,** the top layer after spinning. Plasma is the liquid part of your blood. It acts as a delivery agent, allowing the solid parts of your blood (white cells, platelets, and red blood cells) to **suspend** within it as it travels to all parts of your body. Plasma is about 90% water and salts, but the other 10% is **protein.**

The protein adds density to the plasma and helps the cellular blood parts stay **suspended**. Plasma is yellowish in color. When we give patients additional plasma with a plasma **transfusion**, we must match the patient's and the plasma **donor**'s blood type to avoid an allergic response. Since the proteins play a key role along with platelets in stopping the bleeding from an injury to a blood vessel, we might give our patient plasma if they have a blood **clotting** abnormality.

Platelets and white blood cells remain together in the middle band as you can see in the picture. Think about why they stay together during the spinning process?

Platelets are the reason you don't bleed to death when you get a paper cut. Platelets clump together to form a blood clot when platelets sense they have come into contact with a break in a blood vessel. We can give a platelet transfusion to a patient having a very low platelet count in their blood to prevent bleeding.

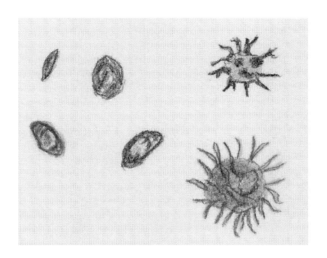

Unlike plasma and red blood cells, platelets do not have a blood type, so they can be transfused freely regardless of blood type. **Hemophilia** is a disease where certain blood **clotting** proteins, also called clotting **factors**, are missing from the plasma; these patients have to be very careful and also receive treatment so they don't bleed to death.

White blood cells provide our bodies with its natural defense against infection or exposure to **toxins** or **allergens**. There are five types of white blood cells found in our blood, but they work together to protect us.

Monocytes are the largest white cells. They are immediate fighters of infection.

Medical Investigation 101

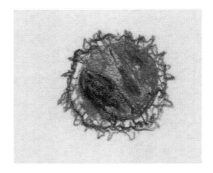

Lymphocytes are our main 'immunity' cells. They recognize and provide a sustained attack on foreign substances such as bacteria and allergens.

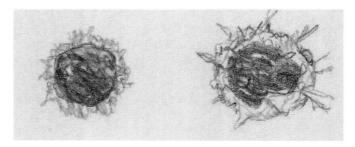

Neutrophils are the most abundant white cell, usually between 40-70 percent of all white cells in your blood. They represent your body's first line of defense against infection.

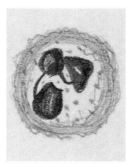

Eosinophils send signals to other white cells telling them to attack. Our blood level of eosinophils goes up when we have an infection or allergy attack.

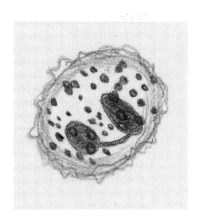

Basophils have two important jobs: first, they prevent blood from clotting too quickly. If our blood started clotting too much whenever we cut ourselves, we would have blood clots flowing through our bodies. It wouldn't take long for a blood clot to move to our lungs and block the flow of blood. We wouldn't survive long in that condition. Basophils also promote the flow of blood into the area needing help by enlarging the size of the small arteries in the region of the body. If you have an infection in your foot, your basophils will send more blood there, bringing along all of the white cells needed to fight the infection.

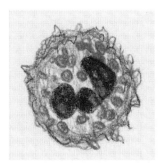

Red blood cells carry **oxygen** to every cell in our body. Also called **erythrocytes**, they make up about half of the total blood **volume** and are the most common blood cell.

Medical Investigation 101

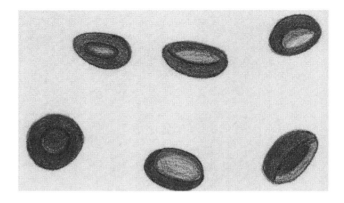

Erythrocytes utilize **hemoglobin** to pick up oxygen in the lungs and deliver it to tissues throughout the body, releasing it as the cells pass through the **capillaries**. The hemoglobin inside the erythrocytes gives these blood cells their red color and their easier-to-remember name "red blood cells." As the red blood cells give up their oxygen they pick up **carbon dioxide** (a waste product of chemical energy production in the cells) from the tissues and return it to the lungs, where it is released when you **exhale.** Before you give a patient a blood transfusion you should know their blood type to avoid an allergic reaction, and indeed hospitals do several tests on blood before a transfusion to make sure you can safely administer it to a specific patient.

Sometimes children are born with abnormal hemoglobin in their red blood cells. Look at the picture above to see the shape of a normal red blood cell. In children born with **Sickle Cell Anemia**, some of their red blood cells under certain situations of stress no longer remain round because of their abnormal hemoglobin. If under stress their red cells become elongated they will not pass through capillaries easily and the patient will develop severe pain from lack of oxygen delivery to specific organs or regions of the body. (Look at the drawing of red blood cells. Do you see the sickled red blood cells among the normally shaped cells?

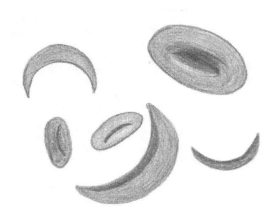

Red Blood Cells of Sickle Cell Anemia patient

Can you see why they call it "Sickle Cell" Anemia?

Investigation 3.5

3.5A: Emergencies
3.5B: Chest Pain

Investigation 3.5A: Emergencies

We have pushed you into the role of a medical doctor taking care of patients who come to you for treatment of their symptoms. You have probably felt some anxiety and tension in filling that role. In this section we want to step back and allow you to play yourself but give you an opportunity to think about medical emergencies that may actually take place in your life. Can we take some of the things you have learned and apply them in that context?

One of the authors of this workbook has grandchildren, two boys, in the early years of elementary school. They were playing by themselves in the basement of their home after getting home from school. A large portion of the basement has been set aside for their play that often seems to center on space travel. They have spaceship models and fictional space character figures based on movies. On this particular afternoon play got vigorous and one of the boys injured himself sufficiently to disrupt the play. His brother raced to the bottom of the stairs and yelled up to his parents, "Medic! Medic!" Perhaps they have seen too many war movies, because the usual cry for help has become, "Medic."

The boys in this story were fine, but all of us have the potential of being involved in a real emergency situation, and almost everyone has a feeling of inadequacy when such an event comes along. This book was never intended by itself to turn you into a healthcare provider, and even the ability to handle common household emergencies may require considerable training and experience. We can still, however, plant a few concepts into your mind here to make you more competent in the face of an actual emergency.

You may find this subject compelling enough to want to actually take a course and earn a certification in **Basic Life Support**. The **American Heart Association** has found that individuals as young as 9 years of age can learn and effectively administer life-saving skills. The **Red Cross** has a certification in emergency skills for young adults who specifically wish to do baby- sitting.

The first basic concept important in every **emergency** we actually demonstrated earlier in our introduction. **Get help**. No matter how much knowledge or skill you have you still need help to deal with a real emergency. Help brings manpower, equipment, medications, and usually transportation to a medical facility if the emergency warrants. The most effective route to getting help usually lies in telephoning **911** or recruiting someone to make that call.

Individuals who have no emergency training frequently feel they can help by getting the victim up, either sitting or on their feet. Fight that impulse. Only move someone injured or stricken if staying put would create more injury, for example, if they have fallen in a room on fire.

The letters **ABC** where originally used in Basic Life Support to focus attention on creating an open **Airway**, getting air to move into the lungs by **Breathing**, and moving oxygen throughout the body via the **Circulation** of blood. That makes good sense if you are thinking that getting oxygen to the brain and heart constitutes the primary objective of **Basic Life Support**. More recent research has changed that thinking to **CAB**. The first objective lies in maintaining circulation of the blood. You will easily remember that when you understand why.

The cells in our body need oxygen to release energy from food to keep you alive, but in the absence of oxygen they can release energy by an alternative chemical reaction for a while. The alternative chemical reaction produces **lactic acid** that can become **toxic** to the cell if it builds up. If the circulation of blood continues the lactic acid will become **diluted** in the blood and delay that toxicity usually long enough to get help. So, if the victim lacks a **pulse,** Basic Life Support procedures now call for vigorous **chest compressions** without stopping to keep the blood moving. The chest compressions take priority over all other steps until help arrives and helps open up additional options for treatment.

Emergency victims who are **bleeding** need prompt attention to stop the loss of blood. Commonly bleeding can be slowed or stopped with **pressure** applied directly to the site of bleeding or to the vessels close to the bleeding.

Healthcare providers once thought we should give fluids to people who were bleeding or elevate arms or legs to raise the blood pressure while moving the patient to a hospital where the bleeding could be stopped. We now know that trying to keep the blood pressure close to normal in patients who are still bleeding actually makes the situation worse. The current recommended strategy lies in applying direct pressure to the wound or vessels as best one can, but, getting the patient to the hospital as quickly as possible without trying to raise the patient's blood pressure before transporting. At the hospital the **surgeons** will rush to stop the bleeding and then the **transfusion** of blood from the **Blood Bank** can begin to restore the blood pressure. Some have called this strategy of getting injured patients to the hospital as quickly as possible without trying to treat them at the scene of injury by the phrase **"Scoop and Run."**

Basic Life Support courses cover what to do in the case of a **heart attack** (chest pain or sudden loss of pulse), a **stroke** (sudden development of weakness, loss of vision, or impaired speech), **choking** (something blocking the passage of air to the lungs), **loss of breathing** (no effective **respiration** or chest movement), and severe **bleeding**. We once had little we could do for a stroke, but now a number of **therapies** can reverse or minimize the effects of stroke if the victim gets to a stroke center quickly. The original time limit for stroke treatment was less than three hours; now some centers allow a longer window; but getting to treatment sooner produces better results.

An emergency that can occur when we don't chew our food adequately, take enormous bites, or just swallow wrong, we call **choking**. Choking can also occur when small children place household objects in their mouths. Choking is an emergency because it physically blocks oxygen from making its way into our **trachea** and traveling to our lungs. Without oxygen in our lungs our vital organs, especially our brain, go into panic mode. Within four minutes of blocking our airway with food or other objects our brain can suffer irreversible damage.

You can tell when someone is choking because they flail about, usually placing their hands to their throat, but not voicing any sounds. They cannot speak because no air can escape from their trachea; we only voice sounds when we exhale air across our vocal chords. Choking victims cannot **exhale**.

So, what should you do if you encounter a friend, a family member, even a stranger who demonstrates the signs of choking? First, ask if they are choking. They will not answer but will probably shake their head up and down. If they answer with a normal voice, they are not choking. When you are convinced they indeed are choking, you can help them using the **Heimlich Maneuver**. Dr. Heimlich proposed this method to expel a blockage of the main stem bronchus (the wind pipe) by squeezing the victim's abdomen. The American Heart Association denounced his method for more than a decade before quietly adding it to their teachings as the scientific evidence grew of its benefits. You can learn this maneuver as part of a basic life support class or perhaps look at http://www.wikihow.com/Perform-the-Heimlich-Maneuver and become an expert.

You can learn basic life support skills and potentially save the life of a family member or friend by knowing how to respond to an emergency before help arrives. You can look up a course on the Internet and perhaps talk a family member into taking one of these courses with you. It is reassuring to know that someone else in the family can help you should the need arise.

The Red Cross and the American Heart Association are two organizations active in most communities that teach emergency response skills.

An extra tip:

We have all heard about heart attacks and know they are quite serious. Our hearts are made of muscle and that muscle works throughout our life pumping blood through our arteries and veins. It never gets a holiday. The term "heart attack" lacks specificity so doctors normally use another term on written records. If arteries that take blood to a region of heart muscle become blocked, those muscle cells with no blood circulation will not have the oxygen and nutrients they need to keep working. If that situation persists those muscle cells will die and physicians call that situation a **myocardial infarction** or an MI.

Usually an MI results from a clot forming in an artery in the heart that blocks the blood flow. Nerve endings in the heart can sense a lack of oxygen. These nerve endings we call **ischemia receptors**, ischemia meaning inadequate oxygen. These receptors cause the sensation we perceive as chest pain, often described as "crushing" in nature. The pain often seems to go into the left arm or up into the neck and jaw. In addition to pain, the receptors increase the rate of heart beats and increase blood pressure by causing the release of hormones that direct arteries to squeeze down (pinch), cutting off blood flow going to **non-vital** organs. When the heart beats faster and has to push the blood through pinched arteries, the heart actually must work harder than before. So, when a patient has chest pain the body actually makes the situation worse by its response to the ischemic receptors making the effected straining muscle not getting enough oxygen work even harder. Emergency physicians give patients with ischemic heart pain medicines that will undo the bad effects caused by these receptors.

You might ask yourself, why would we have a nerve receptor in our body that essentially tries to kill us during a heart attack? If our body evolved traits that made us smarter and stronger over thousands of years, how did this bad trait get there? A number of theories have been proposed. Perhaps the tribe would see an advantage to killing off its older members. That seems very harsh. Another theory suggests that ischemic receptors actually do the right things if the ischemia comes from blood loss rather than a blocked artery. Perhaps we evolved these receptors for instances where tigers attacked and bit cavemen. Consider yet another possibility. The cheetah chases the antelope for less than 30 seconds and then stops before that high-speed chase does damage to the cheetah's heart. Zoologists believe the signal for the cheetah to stop the chase comes from its cardiac ischemic receptors. Perhaps humans got those receptors in the process of evolution before they actually became humans, sort of leftover genes. In any case, it is interesting to think about how our physiology evolved and why.

Also included in that non-specific category of "heart attacks" you will find **ventricular fibrillation**. Ventricular fibrillation, or V-Fib, occurs when the heart muscle's cells become disorganized and no longer beat in the normal sequence that makes the heart an effective blood pump. V-Fib can come from insufficient heart blood flow, but also from other causes (for example, an accident in which electrical current passes through the body). If the heart muscle cells in V-Fib just beat individually any time they want to beat, the heart squirms about but does not actually pump. V-Fib causes **sudden cardiac death,** meaning the patient may have no warning from chest pain, but simply falls down with no pulse. These patients do benefit from chest compression and prompt application of an electrical **defibrillator**, a device currently available in many public buildings and carried about by community emergency response teams. The defibrillator can restore the **coordinated** beat of the muscle cells of the heart when it arrives promptly. This device has saved many lives. The defibrillators in public buildings have a **voice track** that instructs people trying to help how to correctly shock the victim back to life.

Investigation 3.5B: Chest Pain

As many as one quarter of all U.S. citizens may experience chest pain at one time or another. Over five million emergency room visits each year relate to chest pain. Even though the patient may feel certain a heart attack is in progress, not all chest pain comes from a heart attack; of course, a cardiac cause must be ruled out before the patient leaves the emergency room. Fortunately, more than half of the complaints of chest pain in the emergency room end up having another cause unrelated to the heart.

The Mayo Clinic classifies chest pain into five major categories: heart, digestive, bone and muscle, lung, and other. Let's take a look at each of these categories.

As we have discussed, cardiac causes of chest pain include myocardial infarction, angina, aortic dissection, and pericarditis. **A myocardial infarction** requires immediate treatment. Death (infarction means death) of part of the heart muscle results from a blockage to one or more of the arteries within the heart that supply oxygen to the muscle. That blockage can occur suddenly, but often occurs slowly as injuries to the walls of arteries heal by building up a coating called a plaque. As arteries become narrowed by plaque they deliver less blood flow and oxygen. The low flow stimulates the ischemic receptors to create a perception of pain that we call **Angina.** Patients experience angina especially during strenuous activities when the heart needs increased oxygen that the narrowed arteries cannot supply.

The aorta, the body's largest artery, carries the oxygenated blood leaving the heart going to the rest of the body. **Aortic dissection** describes a rupture of this vital structure. Such a tear or rupture can result in an almost sudden death. Before such a rupture occurs the wall of the aorta commonly weakens over time, and its diameter enlarges. Symptoms may not occur until the wall starts to leak blood or suddenly breaks open. Fortunately, some aortic dissections do leak first and thus create discomfort before rupturing, and that allows surgeons an opportunity to repair the leak.

Pericarditis occurs when the protective sac or membrane surrounding the heart, called the **pericardium**, becomes infected or inflamed, Pericarditis may produce pain similar to angina or a myocardial infarction. An inflamed pericardial sac can leak fluid (a fluid similar to the serum portion of blood) into the area around the heart and that fluid can mechanically impede the heart's ability to pump blood.

All cardiac origins of chest pain call for immediate care. But as noted earlier, not all chest pain occurs due to heart problems.

Chest pain commonly occurs in disorders of the digestive system, primarily from the esophagus, gall bladder, or pancreas. **Heartburn** occurs when acid backwashes from the stomach and burns or irritates the inside of the esophagus. The esophagus conveys the food you eat from your mouth to your stomach. Inflammation of the **gall bladder** or **pancreas** located in the abdomen can produce pain that we say "**radiates**" into the chest. As the human body develops before birth these abdominal organs form initially high in the chest and migrate down into the abdomen taking with them the nerves that convey pain from inflammation. The brain still perceives that pain as coming from the chest even though the organ left that location during fetal development.

Disorders of bones and muscles surrounding the chest cavity can certainly cause chest pain. Bruised or broken **ribs**, inflammation of the **cartilage** joining your ribs to the sternum, called **costochondritis**, and injury to the **muscles** of the rib cage can all cause chest pain.

Besides the heart, the lungs reside in the chest. When evaluating chest pain, a thorough evaluation of the lungs makes sense. We must rule out a pulmonary embolism, collapsed lung, pulmonary hypertension, and pleurisy. **Pulmonary embolism** occurs when a blood clot or other foreign material becomes lodged in a lung artery, making it difficult for the lung to exchange gases. A **collapsed lung** can occur spontaneously or due to injury when air leaks out of the lung or through the chest wall into the space between the lung and ribs. As more air leaks out into the space around the lung it becomes more and more difficult to breathe. **Pulmonary hypertension** occurs when the pressure in the arteries traveling to the lungs is above normal, a condition that can cause fluid to accumulate in the lung tissue. **Pleurisy** occurs when the membrane covering of the lungs becomes inflamed, making it painful to expand the lung during **inspiration**.

In addition to the definitive disorders involving the organs and body systems in and around the chest, other non-specific origins of chest pain can occur. Individuals can experience sever stress to a degree that makes them feel ill with chest and abdominal symptoms. **Panic attacks** fall into this category. Such attacks can create chest pain or tightness, rapid heartbeat, air hunger, and other symptoms similar to symptoms seen from a cardiac condition. Pain in the chest wall can also be experienced with an attack of **shingles,** a condition arising from a reactivation of the virus that previously caused a case of chicken pox.

Now you can appreciate the difficulty of managing an extremely agitated patient with chest pain. Although the list of possible causes might stretch one's imagination, and even though you may need to act quickly to avoid rapidly worsening symptoms, your job remains the same. You must rule out potential causes until the one valid explanation remains for you to treat. The stakes in unraveling this puzzle efficiently can easily represent life or death. Welcome to emergency medicine!

Investigation 3.6

3.6A: Chronic Disease

3.6B: Diabetes

Investigation 3.6A: Chronic Disease

Referrals are an important tool within your practice of medicine.

No one knows everything, so a good physician will recognize the limits of his or her abilities, both in knowledge and experience. Other physicians will refer patients to you because they believe you can handle the patient's condition more efficiently. By the same token, you will have patients whom you realize require **expertise** beyond your knowledge and experience; and you will refer those patients to a colleague whom you respect. The next case represents an example of referrals working in both directions for the same patient.

Many of the citizens of our country have a huge problem with **obesity**, so we hear a lot about various **diets** to attack this problem. You probably know that our foods contain three primary components: **protein, fat,** and **carbohydrates**. **Diabetes** is a disease related to the inability to get broken-down carbohydrates, called **glucose**, into the tissues throughout our body. We will talk more about that later.

Diabetes is important in this case because uncontrolled diabetes can inhibit healing following surgery. In this lesson you have a patient named Gilbert who has bad knees. You sent Gilbert to see a surgeon to treat his knees, but the surgeon wants Gilbert to come back to see you. Let's see what happens.

Chief Complaint: You are having a very busy day in your **primary care** office, seeing all sorts of patients, non-stop, when your receptionist pulls you away to take a phone call from an **orthopedic surgeon** in your community. When you take Dr. Drazer's call, she jumps right over any small talk and goes right to the issue.

"I've got your patient Gilbert Isaacs with me here in the office and as you thought he needs a new left knee sooner rather than later." You referred Gilbert to Dr. Drazer only a few days ago because his knee pain had stopped responding to your **conservative treatment regimen**. People generally stay healthier when they are active in some way every day and Gilbert's knee pain had gotten so bad he had become a fixture on a couch.

"Well I am delighted that you can help him," you respond. Dr. Drazer, who must also have her office full of patients, shot right back, "But Gilbert has a **hemoglobin A1c** of 7.8 drawn yesterday, and I need him lower than 6 for a week before I dare put a **steel knee** into his leg. Can you get him there for me and keep me informed so I can work him into the **surgery schedule** as quickly as possible?" Without even waiting for my response she added, "I'll have him call your office and come in to see you. Thanks for sending him to me." The phone went "click" in my ear. I guess I had a new chief complaint, not from the patient, but from the patient's surgeon.

Review of Medical Records: Gilbert Isaacs is a 72-year-old male, retired businessman. He has been in your care for the past twelve years. When you were introduced to Gilbert he was very overweight, weighing in at 270 pounds. Gilbert mentioned at his annual physical exam eleven years ago that for the past year he experienced getting up eight to ten times during the night to urinate and that he had recently lost a significant amount of weight in a short period of time without dieting. Gilbert thought this was a normal result of drinking a lot of water due to extreme thirst. This history had prompted you to perform a series of blood tests that had confirmed the diagnosis. Gilbert demonstrated elevated levels of blood glucose starting about 10 years ago, and a **glucose tolerance test** confirmed the diagnosis back then of **Type II Diabetes**. Since that time Gilbert maintained a **low carbohydrate diet** (a diet popularly known as the Adkin's Diet) and two years ago he started taking a pill that decreases the production of glucose by the liver. Gilbert has never taken insulin shots.

Since that time, he has returned twice each year for evaluation of his diabetic status and adjustment of his oral medication. However, over the past six months you have seen him in the office more frequently concerning swelling and pain in his left knee. You have prescribed oral anti-inflammatory medicines and referred him for physical therapy over the past several months without benefit to the patient. Last week you referred him to Dr. Drazer for an **orthopedic consultation**. He is now referred back for control of his **diabetes** so that he can undergo surgical replacement of his severely arthritic left knee with a **prosthetic knee**.

Dr. Drazer has asked that Gilbert's hemoglobin A1c stay below 6 for a week. This request comes from an observation that levels above 6 predict a significantly higher incidence of infections following joint replacement surgery. An infection in an artificial joint proves very difficult to resolve, unless the surgeon actually removes the artificial joint so that antibiotic medications reach the infection. No one wants to go through that process. When patients have an elevated glucose over an extended period of time the glucose attaches to the proteins in the patient's blood stream and that causes the ability of white blood cells to fight infections to diminish. So, it is not enough to simply get the blood glucose level down to normal on the day of surgery, Dr. Drazer needs the serum glucose level down to normal levels for a week or more to make sure the white cells have returned to their normal infection fighting capabilities.

Examination:

    Height, 5' 11, **Weight**: 188 pounds

    Blood Pressure is 132/89. **Pulse** = 122 b/min   **Temperature** (Oral) = 98.6 F.

    Head and Neck:

    Eyes: vision corrected with glasses, **trifocals**

    Ears: normal examination

    Mouth: **partial denture**, otherwise normal

    Neck: normal anatomy, no **carotid bruits**

    Heart: normal sounds, no sign of **cardiac** enlargement, normal **sinus rhythm**

    Lungs: breathe sounds normal all quadrants

Abdomen: **bowel sounds** active, no masses or tenderness, no **liver distention**, no **renal** discomfort on **percussion**

Extremities: enlarged left knee with reduced range of motion and significant discomfort on both extension and flexion.

Reflexes and **pulses** normal.

Differential Diagnosis: For this particular patient there is no differential diagnosis. You are fully aware of Gilbert's diagnoses:

       a. Type II Diabetes, not well controlled

       b. Arthritis left knee with a recommendation of knee replacement

Medical Tests

Below is a summary of some available tests to consider and a short description of how they might help your medical investigation:

Think about which test(s) would be most appropriate at this time? (write down any that apply)

- **CBC (complete blood count)**
- **Random Plasma Glucose**
- **Magnetic Resonance Image (MRI)** of pancreas and liver
- **Hemoglobin A1C** blood test
- **Ultrasound** of pancreas and liver
- **X-Ray** of Abdomen

Immediate Treatment Options:

Look at the list of potential treatments and decide which would be most appropriate for your patient while waiting for test results:

Medical Investigation 101

- **Emergency Surgery** to remove the pancreas and/or liver.
- **Radiation therapy** to stimulate the pancreas to produce more insulin.
- **Prescription** for stronger insulin stimulating medicine
- **Prescription** for insulin and needles
- **No change of prescriptions** until all tests come back with results.

Test results:

Since Gilbert is already known to have type II diabetes, the appropriate test would be the Hemoglobin A1C. This test tells you Gilbert's average blood glucose over the past two to three months. This is very helpful in letting you know how well Gilbert has been controlling his disease.

Complete Blood Count (CBC)	Analyzes the amount of red blood cells, white blood cells, and platelets in blood sample
Random Plasma Glucose	Provides blood glucose level at any point in time from small blood specimen
Magnetic Resonance Imaging (MRI)	Provides a layer by layer view of the pancreas and liver
Hemoglobin A1C Blood Test	Provides an index of average blood glucose over past 2-3 month timeframe by measuring glucose bound to protein hemoglobin in the blood sample
Ultrasound of Pancreas & Liver	Uses sound to visualize the structures of the pancreas and liver
X-Ray of Abdomen	Shows the spine and any areas of calcification of the pancreas or liver

The following chart represents the key to reading Hemoglobin A1C test results:

Diabetes Diagnosis	Hemoglobin A1C level in blood
Normal (non-diabetic)	Less than (<) 5.7%
Pre-diabetic	Between 5.7% and 6.4%
Diabetes	6.5% or greater

Gilbert's Hemoglobin A1C test comes back with a result of 7.8%. What is the current state of his diabetic disease? Think about which of the following you would write on this patient's chart for the current assessment of his diabetes?

    Normal   Pre-Diabetic   Diabetic
    Well controlled diabetes   Out of control diabetes

You now have to consider whether Gilbert is a good candidate to be referred back to Dr. Drazer for knee surgery in the next week? Think about what you might tell Dr. Drazer when you call to report your findings.

Additional food for thought:

Type II (the Roman numeral we read as two) **Diabetes** has become all too common in our population. Normally, special islands of cells in the **pancreas** (a long, slender organ just under the stomach) monitor the level of sugar in our bloodstream. If we eat sugar and the sugar level goes too high, the cells in the pancreas **excrete** insulin into the bloodstream to ask all the cells in the body to take more sugar molecules inside and use that sugar for energy to drive the cells' activities. On the other hand, if we do not eat any sugar, those same cells in the pancreas release another **hormone** to encourage the **liver** to convert some of its stored carbohydrates back into glucose. In Type II Diabetes the patient makes insulin, but the cells throughout our body have become ineffective in **absorbing** more **glucose** when called upon to do so. Patients with Type II Diabetes (sometimes called **insulin resistant** diabetes) generally have a **progressive** chronic disease course treated first by reducing sugar in their diet, next with pills that make insulin more effective, and finally they may need to get insulin by **injection** or **inhalation** (currently an experimental method of administration). You cannot absorb **insulin** through your stomach or intestines because the normal digestive process our bodies use treats insulin (a protein) as food and tears it apart (digestion) for use in building new proteins inside our cells.

Type I Diabetes shares the same problem of elevated blood glucose, but in this case the problem lies completely in the pancreas with the cells that make the insulin. Those cells have been destroyed in Type I Diabetes by the body's natural defenses to a viral infection. We see Type I Diabetes occurring generally in children and young adults who appear to have a **genetic abnormality** that allows the virus to produce this effect. We say those patients are "**insulin dependent**" because they must receive daily doses of insulin by injections or inhalation in order to live.

Medical Investigation 101

Types III, IV, and V Diabetes exist but you can put off learning about them until you get to medical school.

Investigation 3.6B: Diabetes

Now that you know how **diabetes** can prevent patients from effectively receiving treatment for other problems, let's take a look at some big picture concerns we as physicians have about our diabetic patients. Why should we be so concerned? The prevalence of diabetes is growing, not just in the United States, but also around the world. It has been estimated that nearly one in four Americans now have diabetes; and the incidence continues to grow in every part of the world.

Sadly, **obesity** has increased even faster than diabetes. It has been shown that obesity significantly increases your patient's chances of becoming a Type II Diabetic; that is a person who develops diabetes later in life rather than someone born with a malfunctioning pancreas (Type 1 Diabetes).

America has a very diverse population, with people from many different places and cultures. In case you are wondering which of your patients have the greatest risk of developing diabetes based on their **ethnicity**, studies have shown that about 16% of Native Americans have diabetes, followed by about 13% of blacks and Hispanics, 9% of Asian Americans, and finally around 7.5% of whites.

You understand that Diabetes does not affect all ethnicities equally. Think about some of the factors of different **cultures** that might affect their risk of diabetes.

Because **diet** is so important in promoting Type II Diabetes, for most people the disease is entirely **preventable**. When we look at ethnic cultures having high rates of diabetes we can look at their diets and analyze what they eat. We can then compare their dietary differences to cultures suffering less diabetes and similarities to cultures also having higher rates of diabetes. We have learned that certain **dietary practices** influence your patients' chances of coming to your office with the symptoms of diabetes; there are also lifestyle changes you can recommend to help prevent your patients from ever suffering the

complications of diabetes. Look at the chart below. It demonstrates some healthy lifestyle factors that can prevent the onset of Diabetes.

Prevention of Diabetes Complications

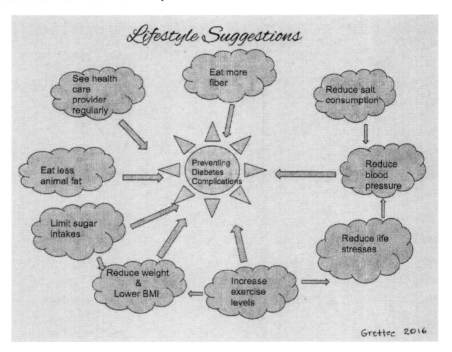

Many of the **preventive measures** listed above relate to diet and regular activity. But you must be prepared for those patients who are not willing to change their habits to a healthier lifestyle. Let's face it; change is difficult. One of the most important roles you will have as a physician is that of an **educator**; yes, you will spend a great deal of time teaching your patients how to live a healthier life. Just like in school, not all of your patients will take your advice. That is the reason you will see many patients suffering the effects of poorly controlled diabetes over many years. Diabetes affects many areas of the body. Look at the following chart to see the many areas that are affected.

Diabetes Complications

All of these complications are very serious to your patient's health. Your diabetic patients will spend more time in the hospital and live shorter, less fulfilling lives than most of your other patients. Heart disease from diabetes makes the heart become less efficient at pumping blood to the rest of the body. Extra **glucose** in the blood injures the kidneys and damages the **capillary** blood flow to the small vessels and nerves, causing **neuropathy, retinopathy,** and **gangrene.**

Diabetes effects the entire body.

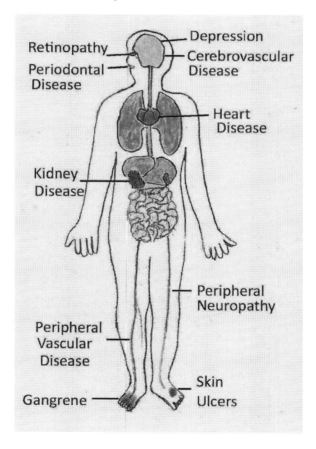

Medical Investigation 101

Diabetic Retinopathy of the Eye

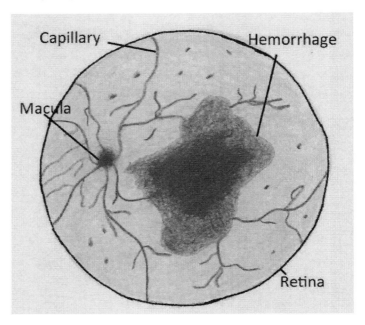

The **retina** is the area of the eye that acts like a movie screen. Diabetes over time injures the walls of the small blood vessels in the eye, and they become prone to rupture and bleeding. When blood **hemorrhages** from the small vessels of the retina, it's like watching a movie with a large ink spot on the screen; you can't see anything in that area. Patients may gradually lose their ability to read or watch TV. The damage to the retina from bleeding can be seen by looking in your patient's eyes using an **ophthalmoscope,** as seen in the drawing of the retina.

Diabetes similarly damages small blood vessels elsewhere, especially the feet, where gravity tends to make the pressure inside vessels higher than other parts of the body. The Diabetic patient may develop ulcers and even gangrene as shown below. Gangrene occurs when the tissues (skin and muscle) die. The dead tissue must be removed, even if it's an entire toe, or worse yet, an entire lower half of the leg.

Diabetic Foot Complications

Diabetic patients have very fragile skin caused by poor circulation and lack of nerve sensation. Ulcers may occur on a toe.

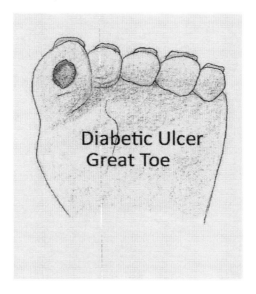

Diabetic skin ulcers also can occur on the leg, or any place on the body subject to pressure on the skin.

Medical Investigation 101

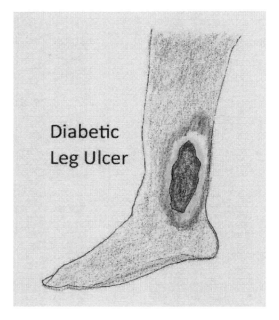

Should diabetes narrow arteries and restrict the blood supply so severely that the tissue cannot survive, gangrene (cell death) occurs.

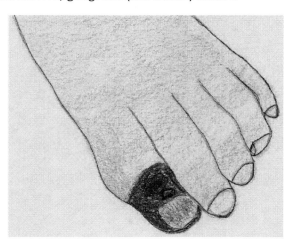

Now you understand why it is so important that you stress healthy eating, regular activity, and weight control for your patients? Otherwise, you may spend a lot of time with them treating the complications of their diabetes, even having to visit them too often in the hospital. Let's take a closer look at how our body uses and regulates glucose.

Abdominal Organs near Pancreas

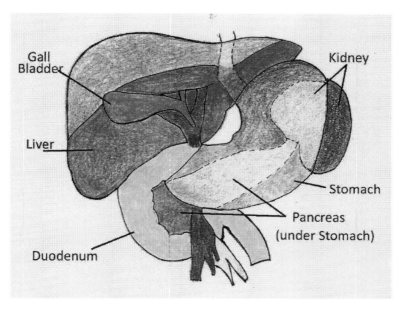

The pancreas is the long, slender area lying mostly under the stomach in the figure above. Its job involves keeping the amount of circulating glucose, a form of sugar our body utilizes, within a controlled range. It is important to treat your pancreas with respect by eating a good diet, exercising, and controlling your weight. Without proper regulation of glucose by insulin and glucagon our bodies seem to fall apart rather quickly. The accepted normal range for glucose in our blood is between 80 and 120 mg/dL (milligrams per deciliter). The level is usually lowest in the morning before breakfast and highest after eating.

The pancreas has two types of specialized cells located in an area called the **Islets of Langerhans**, named after the scientist who discovered them. **Beta cells** release **insulin** when the blood sugar gets too high; insulin increases absorption of glucose into all the cells in the body and thus lowers blood sugar to the normal range. On the other hand, if the blood sugar gets too low, the **Alpha cells** give off **glucagon**, which tells the liver to convert stored glycogen into glucose and release it to raise the blood sugar. So basically, insulin lowers blood sugar and glucagon raises blood sugar. Medical technology may evolve to make pancreatic transplants to treat diabetes. Alternatively, researchers may develop artificial systems that will replace the function of the pancreas. For now, it is important to treat your pancreas with respect by eating a good diet, exercising, and controlling your weight; without proper regulation of glucose by insulin and glucagon our bodies seem to fall apart rather quickly.

Investigation 3.7

3.7A: Shoulder Pain

3.7B: Joints

Investigation 3.7A: Shoulder Pain

When your staff schedules an appointment, they ask the patient the nature of the problem and estimate the amount of time you will need to deal with the issues. Most of your appointments involve a sickness, but sometimes an injury prompts the visit.

Physicians commonly classify an injury according to the duration of symptoms as acute, sub-acute, or chronic. **Acute** injuries occurred very recently, usually in the past few days. An athlete visiting you because he or she injured an ankle playing volleyball yesterday is experiencing an <u>acute</u> injury. **Sub-acute** injuries occurred less recently, perhaps from a few weeks up to a couple months ago. We classify injuries as **chronic** when they occurred months ago, but still produce **symptoms**. The duration of symptoms impacts the strategy for assessment and care. Acute injuries commonly require more diagnostics tests, while sub-acute and chronic injuries dictate a greater focus on therapeutic **modalities**. All injuries begin as acute injuries; for acute injuries you hope to heal the injury to avoid sub-acute or chronic symptoms.

Chief Complaint: George is a 67-year-old male with a chief complaint of right shoulder pain.

History of Chief Complaint:

George reports his pain has been present for at least six months. He does not recall a specific injury that **precipitated** the pain. The pain started as mild and **intermittent** in the right shoulder area, but for the past two months it has become almost constant during his waking hours and occasionally severe on movement of the shoulder. To get relief he takes an over-the-counter **anti-inflammatory** medication once or twice every three days. However, the pain keeps coming back.

When you ask George to describe the pain, he says he feels it mostly at the top of the shoulder, but sometimes he notices pain also at the front or back of the shoulder. Sometimes he gets temporary relief by pressing on the back of his shoulder. He describes the pain occasionally as very intense for a short period of time, up to 9/10 on the **pain scale**. His pain makes it difficult to shave, brush his teeth, and hold a full glass of water. He definitely feels pain and also feels some weakness. He experiences pain when he lies down to sleep, having great difficulty finding a comfortable position for his shoulder.

George has retired from a career as a salesman. His sales position did not include heavy lifting. His current exercise comes from walking, but he enjoyed playing baseball until the age of 54. Indeed, George reports he had quite a reputation on the mound as a strong right-handed pitcher. He still enjoys bowling on occasion, again right-handed.

George reports his past medical history includes surgeries for **appendicitis** at age 14 and removal of a **cyst** from his left wrist about age 37. George has been taking medications for **hypertension** and borderline **diabetes** for several years. He is right side **dominant**, as noted above.

Current Medications:

Metformin 400 mg **Bid**

Lisinopril 20 mg **QD**

Naproxen Sodium 220 mg BID **prn**

Examination:

Temperature: 98.6 F.

Blood Pressure: 145/82

Head and Neck: within normal limits

Heart and Lungs: within normal limits

Abdomen: within normal limits

Upper Extremities: left and right muscular and **osseous symmetry**. Right shoulder tender to **palpation anterior, posterior, superior** and **lateral** areas. **Mobilization** of right shoulder joint **elicits crepitus** and a complaint of increased discomfort. **Splinting** and weakness to **resistance tests** in all **parameters** noted in right shoulder only. Shoulder is stable. No **edema** or **erythema** observed. Left shoulder within normal limits. Normal lower extremities.

Below is the list of possible causes of George's shoulder pain. You can see there are too many possible causes for you to test for every single one. Besides, George would be very unhappy with you if you allowed him to suffer while you worked your way through the entire list. The Differential Diagnosis for Shoulder Pain according to the Mayo Clinic[1] is:

- Avascular necrosis
- Brachial plexus injury
- Broken arm
- Bursitis
- Cervical radiculopathy
- Dislocated shoulder
- Frozen shoulder
- Separated shoulder
- Septic arthritis
- Tendinitis
- Tendon rupture
- Thoracic outlet syndrome
- Torn Cartilage

- Heart attack
- Impingement
- Sprains and strains
- Osteoarthritis
- Polymyalgia rheumatica
- Rheumatoid arthritis
- Rotator cuff injury

Reference:

[1] http://www.mayoclinic.org/symptoms/shoulder-pain/basics/causes/sym-20050696

As George's physician, you must consider every possible cause on the list. However, you feel you can help George more if you rule out the least likely causes right away and quickly arrive at a "**working differential diagnosis**" of the most likely causes. In order to eliminate unlikely causes of George's shoulder pain you can compare what George told you about his symptoms and your examination findings to the **Differential Diagnosis Versus Symptom Chart** on the next page; the chart indicates which symptoms are more likely to occur in each of the possible causes. Match up as many of George's symptoms to the potential disorders to shorten your differential diagnosis down to the three or four most likely causes. **Write down your most likely culprits** (from the list of possibilities on the next page).

Shoulder Pain Differential Diagnoses versus Symptoms Chart

Shoulder Pain DDX	Acute Onset	Gradual Onset	Unilateral	Bilateral	Single Area	Multiple Areas	Male > Female	Female > Male	Pain Localized	Pain Radiates	Fever	Joint Crepitus	Erythema	Edema
Brachial Plexus Injury	X		X		X				X	X				
Broken Arm	X		X		X				X					X
Cervical Radiculopathy		X	X	X	X	X			X	X				
Dislocated Shoulder	X		X		X				X					X
Frozen Shoulder		X	X		X				X			X		
Heart Attack	X		X		X	X				X				
Osteoarthritis		X	X		X	X	X		X			X		
Rheumatoid Arthritis		X		X		X		X	X		X	X	X	X
Rotator Cuff Injury	X	X	X		X				X					
Separated Shoulder	X		X		X				X					
Septic Arthritis	X		X		X				X		X	X	X	X
Tendonitis	X	X	X		X	X			X			X		
Tendon Rupture	X		X		X				X					X
George's Symptoms														

Medical Investigation 101

Once you reduce your differential diagnosis to a manageable number of possibilities you are ready to consider which tests might help you make your final diagnosis. You have available tests to analyze blood, **x-rays** to look inside the body at bones and joints, **Magnetic Resonance Imaging** (MRI) to evaluate soft tissue structures such as muscles, ligaments, and cartilage. **Computerize Tomography** (CT Scan) is a special X-Ray test that can provide clearer definition of internal anatomy when faced with a difficult diagnostic problem.

When you consider which test you will order first you must also consider how much each test costs. A blood test can range from inexpensive to expensive, depending on the type of information you request. Plain X-ray images are much less expensive than an MRI. An MRI or CT Scan may cost well over $1000. We must always compare the expense versus the helpfulness of the test in reaching a diagnosis.

You will also want to consider the effect on the patient when deciding what test to order. For example, the effect on the body from X-rays accumulates with every x-ray ordered. The risk of developing a cancer from exposure to x-ray radiation increases a little with each x-ray exposure in their lifetime. CT scans utilize large amounts of x-ray radiation. A CT scan on the chest, for example, requires about 15 times the radiation exposure needed for a plain chest x-ray. **Nerve Conduction Velocity tests** of peripheral nerves are expensive and uncomfortable for the patient.

Because of the costs and risks, you have a responsibility to order only those tests that are truly necessary to assist you in making the correct diagnosis.

Tests: Which tests do you want to order for George? You can make a list on paper and number the tests in order from most useful to least important for your assessment of George's shoulder (leave blank the space next to tests you do not need):

- Complete blood count
- x-rays of right shoulder
- X-rays of cervical spine
- X-rays of lumbar spine
- MRI of right shoulder
- CT Scan of right shoulder
- Muscle Grip Strength Testing
- Nerve Conduction Velocity

The following chart contains the results you would receive for each test you selected for George. Just for fun see if the tests you did not select would have been helpful.

Test	Results
Complete Blood Count	All findings within normal limits
x-rays of right shoulder	Severe degenerative changes within the shoulder joint with spurring
x-rays of cervical spine	Mild degenerative changes
x-rays of the lumber spine	No herniation or degenerative changes
MRI right shoulder	Severe degenerative joint changes
CT Scan right shoulder	Severe degenerative joint changes
Muscle Grip Strength Testing	Weakness in right hand vs left hand
Nerve Conduction Velocity Test	Within normal limits

X-rays of the right shoulder would have been a good place to start. You might follow-up with an MRI of that shoulder to gain additional information about the condition of the soft tissue structures.

Here is an example of a normal Anterior/Posterior (AP) x-ray of a right shoulder. A complete set of shoulder x-rays would include three views: AP, lateral (LAT), and oblique views.

Medical Investigation 101

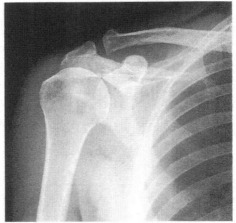

X-ray of normal right shoulder

The next x-ray demonstrates degenerative arthritis of the shoulder joint, as identified by the label "Loss of joint cartilage" and "Osteophyte" labels. Notice the diminished space between the head of the humerus and the glenoid fossa of the scapula when compared to the normal x-ray.

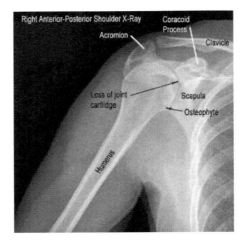

Investigation 3.7B: Joints

All normal bending of our body occurs at **joints**. Whether you straighten your knee, make a circle with your arm, flex your wrist, or turn your head, the bending occurs at one or more joints. Without moveable joints we would essentially be statues.

Our hip and shoulder joints are **ball and socket** joints capable of motion through a range of angles and directions. Flexible hip joints allow us to jump over a hurdle or do splits. Without a ball and socket shoulder joint you could not raise your arm so freely over your head.

Our knees, elbows, fingers, and toes act as **hinge** joints, moving along a single **axis** of **flexion** and **extension**. Flexing the elbow allows you to lift a glass of water to take a drink. Extending your knee allows you to stand up from your chair.

The bones on either side of a moveable joint maintain their connection by way of **ligaments**; without ligaments we would not have the tethering of bones required to create the **leverage** needed to do work. The actual energy for movement comes from the surrounding **muscles**; flexion of the elbows is produced by the **biceps** muscle, while extension is created by the **triceps**.

We also have joints we classify as slightly moveable and non-moveable. Technically a joint occurs wherever two bones meet. In some cases we desire very minimal movement from a joint, such as between the bones of the **spine**. Some joints begin as moveable and, during **maturation**, fuse together, such as the bones of our **skull**. In infancy these bones connect together loosely to allow growth; **fusion** of the bones occurs at the completion of growth when we all become 'hard heads". (Just kidding).

All joints have an enclosure, or boundary, surrounding them, a barrier known as the joint capsule. Within the capsule **lubrication** of the joint surfaces by **synovial fluid** protects the joint surfaces from grinding away the protective **articulating cartilage** surface of bone.

A mechanic puts grease into the "joints' in your parents' automobile for exactly the same purpose. As we reach middle to old age we produce less synovial fluid, often resulting in the **degeneration** of joint surfaces known as **osteoarthritis**. In some unfortunate people their own immune systems attack their joints as if they were foreign invaders, a condition we call **rheumatoid arthritis**.

Healthy and properly functioning joints contribute immensely to our quality of life. Those having unhealthy joints may suffer from the inability to perform even the activities of normal living. They may suffer chronic pain and their inactivity of limitations can lead to depression and even desperation. Restoring joint function and reducing pain and disability are important contributions provided by Orthopedists when they restore quality of life to their patients.

Injuries to bones and joints are often referred to Orthopedic Surgeons for further evaluation and treatment; they specialize in the treatment of injuries and diseases affecting the bones and joints. Orthopedists are the "carpenters of the medical community" who treat patients of all ages with problems with their "skeletal scaffolding". Children might injure bones and joints when they fall off their skateboard or bicycle. Unfortunately, some people are born with bone deformities that require treatment, so-called congenital deformities. Teenagers and young adults may sometimes think they are invincible, driving cars erratically, inviting a crash or getting into fights. Sports injuries can occur even when taking all appropriate precautions. Adults sometimes suffer work related injuries or have accidents. Elderly patients' joints can wear out and require replacement. Almost everyone needs an Orthopedist somewhere along his or her life's journey.

Orthopedic Surgery has several sub-specialties to include surgeons who focus exclusively on the spine, hand, shoulder, hip, lower leg and foot, even non-surgical orthopedic treatments and rehabilitation. Orthopedists who have not completed a fellowship in a sub-specialty are considered General Orthopedists; they treat basic bone or joint problems of a more routine nature. Sub-specialists use their advanced training to manage more complex orthopedic problems referred to them for care.

We can see a good example of orthopedic sub-specialization in the world of professional baseball. Pitchers at that level throwing thousands of baseballs at high velocity are prone to two particular career-limiting injuries: (1) tears of the rotator cuff and labrum of the shoulder and (2) tearing of the ligaments of the elbow. A Major League baseball team would insist their pitcher with the shoulder injury receive treatment from a surgeon who works exclusively on sports injuries to elbow ligaments. Medicine is very specialized in this modern age, where amazingly complex procedures can literally rebuild the injured structure.

Not all patients referred to Orthopedic Surgeons require surgery. In fact, Orthopedists generally reserve surgery as a last resort only recommended when conservative treatments such as rest, medication, therapeutic injections, and physical therapy have failed to resolve pain and restore function. All surgery has a risk of failure or infection and should receive careful and informed consideration. Surgeons themselves often define major surgery as "any surgery done on me".

Orthopedists have an extensive arsenal of options available when surgery becomes necessary. A partial list of procedures often performed by Orthopedists include:

- Closed reduction of a displaced fracture
- Open reduction of a displaced fracture
- Excision and curettage of infected bone and tissue
- Bone Biopsy of suspected bone cancer
- Reattachment of torn muscles or ligaments
- Total joint replacement for arthritis of shoulder, hip, knee, or ankle
- Repair of torn rotator cuff of shoulder
- Ligament replacement in elbow
- Arthroscopic surgery of knee
- Ligament replacement of knee

- Spinal Fusion

Non-surgical orthopedic treatments include application of casts, injections of local anesthetics and steroids, physical mobilization or traction therapy, prescribing oral medications, and many more.

With so many people participating in sports, injured in car accidents, and suffering diseases **afflicting** joints and bones, orthopedists are, indeed, very busy physicians. Orthopedic medicine continues to develop highly technical treatments for orthopedic problems. It is nearly impossible for a single orthopedist to become proficient in all areas of this constantly expanding specialty. Perhaps the value of sub-specialization makes more sense to you now.

Investigation 3.8

3.8A: Fever and Cough
3.8B: The Lungs

Investigation 3.8A: Fever and Cough

Introduction:

Fever and cough are two of the most common complaints you see in your family medicine practice. These two symptoms let you know something is not right with the patient, but fever and cough occur in many illnesses, both acute and chronic. Hearing or seeing these symptoms doesn't take your mind immediately to the source of the problem; rather, they cause you to ask 'Why' does the patient exhibit these symptoms?

How many times in your life would you guess you have asked the question, "Why?" Your parents might say you asked that question a million times, but they might also say that your curiosity about the world made you the special person you have become. Today you must ask lots of questions of a new patient in your office complaining of episodes of fever and a cough, a cough that stubbornly refuses to go away.

Chief Complaint:
"I thought it was just a viral infection that came on about four weeks ago," said 20-year-old, Manjula Mehroul, a business student at the community college in your community. "I just cannot seem to shake it. I am worried that I have mono. Do you really get that from kissing?"

History of Present Illness:
You answer Manjula's question about **mononucleosis**. Mono, a common **viral infection** among college students, can spread through saliva which leads to its slang name, "the kissing disease." Manjula knows people who have mono.

As you listen to Manjula you have mono high on your differential diagnosis list, except a history of cough is usually not part of the normal presentation of mono. You want to ask some basic questions to better understand what has been happening to Manjula. You soon learn that she came to the United States at age 4. Her parents both grew up in India. Manjula can barely remember anything about living in India. However, she has visited her relatives in India. In fact she returned to India two months ago with her parents because her Grandmother had fallen ill and died. Manjula's recent visit to India lasted only a week. Back at school in America, Manjula noted that her schoolwork and study seemed exhausting, much more exhausting than her previous year. In fact, she complained that she could never remember being this tired, and she wondered at first if she somehow had chosen professors who demand excessive work from their students.

You ask Manjula about her complaint of fever and she says that three times she has felt feverish and awakened in the morning feeling damp and sweaty. She added that she had also awakened during the night coughing, and even had violent episodes of coughing during the day. The coughs brought up thick mucus sometimes and once she thought the mucus may have had just a little blood in it.

You also learn that Manjula has never smoked. She does not recall ever having had a headache. She has not had a recent sore throat or any problem with her tonsils or sinuses. She has not had any rash, or swollen lymph glands in her neck, groin, or armpits.

Review of Systems:
A review of systems reveals that she had both **measles** and **chicken pox** as a child. Her parents made sure she got her childhood shots. She had no surgery

ever and had never been in the hospital. She had no problems ever with her heart, lungs, kidneys, stomach, or nervous system.

Medications: none

Allergies: none

Examination:
Wt: 127 lbs.   Respirations: 18 /min   Pulse: 86 /min
Blood Pressure: 122/76   Temperature: 98.8° F.
General: Healthy appearing young female, well developed, well nourished, of Asian dissent, in no acute distress.
Head: No abnormal findings. No enlarged **lymph nodes**. No redness in the ears or throat. Normal range of movement of the neck. No **thyroid** enlargement.
Heart: No abnormal sounds
Lungs: Rhonchi (coarse rattling sound), and deep breaths stimulated coughing episode. Small sample of **sputum** collected.
Abdomen: Soft, no tenderness, normal **bowel sounds**.
Extremities: No deformities. No swelling. No tenderness.

Assessment: Normally healthy and active young woman in no acute distress but appears to have some **respiratory** symptoms and fevers, and a history of **international** travel in the recent past.

Look at the Chart. Compare the symptoms discovered in the history and physical examination to those of the conditions that must be ruled out or confirmed as your investigation leads you toward making your final diagnosis.

Differential Diagnosis Chart:

Look at the following "Hallmark Signs" summary to examine some of the "classic symptoms" of each of the diseases from our list. Compare them to Manjula's symptoms.

Symptoms:

DDX list	Fever	Cough	Lymph Nodes	Fatigue	Mucus/Sputum	Skin Rash	Headaches	Hoarse Voice	Sore Throat	Joint Pain	Acute/Chronic	Weight Loss	Appetite Loss	Rales/Rhonchi	Night Sweats
Mononucleosis	X	X	X	X	X	X	X	X	X	X	A	X	X	X	X
Lung Abscess	X	X	X	X	X	X	X	X	X	X	AC	X	X	X	X
Hodgkin's Lymphoma	X		X	X	X	X		X	X	X	AC	X	X	X	X
Atypical Pneumonia	X	X	X	X	X	X	X	X	X	X	A	X	X	X	X
Lung Tuberculosis	X	X	X	X	X	X	X	X	X	X	AC	X	X	X	X
Sarcoidosis	X	X	X	X	X	X	X	X	X	X	AC	X	X	X	X
Brucellosis	X	X	X	X	X	X	X	X	X	X	AC	X	X	X	X
Blastomycosis	X	X	X	X	X	X	X	X	X	X	AC	X	X		X
Non-Hodgkin's Lymphoma	X	X	X	X	X	X		X	X	X	AC	X	X	X	X
Cat-Scratch Fever	X	X	X	X		X	X	X	X	X	A	X	X	X	X
Lupus Erythematosis	X	X	X	X		X		X	X	X	AC	X	X	X	X
Patient Manjula															

Looking at this differential diagnosis list you likely found unfamiliar names. This is proof that medical science often seems like a foreign language. Just the names of all known diseases takes you well beyond 10,000 words; indeed the number of **genetic diseases** alone experts think exceeds 10,000. You can look up each disease on this list and see how closely that disease fits this particular patient's situation. Hopefully, you noticed the symptoms for all of your choices are very similar. And this is often the physician's dilemma, and the reason that finding the actual diagnosis is often a process of elimination by symptoms and medical tests.

It is important to determine if Manjula's illness is contagious, since we don't want her spreading whatever she has throughout our entire community. So you might ask yourself if this list represents particular categories of disease; and indeed it does, **infectious diseases** and m**alignancies** (cancers). Make a list of the illnesses listed below. Put an **"I"** before each disease that you categorize as infectious and a **"C"** before each disease that you categorize as a cancer in this list:

Hallmark signs:

1. **Mononucleosis**: sore throat, swollen lymph nodes, swollen tonsils, headache or body ache, fatigue, loss of appetite, and pain in the upper left abdominal quadrant (spleen).

2. **Lung Abscess**: fever, cough with foul-smelling sputum, night sweats, appetite loss, and weight loss.

3. **Hodgkin's Lymphoma**: swollen, painless lymph nodes, fevers, fatigue, drenching night sweats, unplanned weight loss, unexplained itching, unexplained low back pain, lymph node pain on consuming alcoholic beverages.

4. **Atypical Pneumonia**: low-grade fever, headache, hacking cough, fatigue, chills, sore throat, chest or stomach pain, appetite loss, vomiting

5. **Lung Tuberculosis**: bad cough lasting more than three weeks, pain in the chest, coughing up blood or sputum, fatigue, appetite loss, weight loss, chills, fever, night sweats.

6. **Sarcoidosis**: wheezing, coughing, shortness of breath, weight loss, night sweats, bone or joint pain, anemia, or no symptoms at all.

7. **Brucellosis**: fever, sweats, appetite loss, headache, muscle ache, joint or back pain, or fatigue

8. **Blastomycosis**: fever, chills, cough, muscle aches, joint pain, and chest pain or no symptoms.

9. **Non-Hodgkin's Lymphoma**: swollen lymph glands, fever, chills, night sweats, itching, weight loss, headaches.

10. **Lung Cancer**: persistent cough that may worsen, chest pain worse with inspiration, coughing, laughing, hoarseness, weight loss, appetite loss, coughing up blood or rust-colored sputum, fatigue, new onset wheezing.

From the history would you expect Manjula has cancer or an infection?

What laboratory studies would you like to conduct? Write down or make a mental list.

- White blood cell count
- Pulmonary function test
- Cultures of the sputum sample obtained
- Chest X-Ray of lung and a PPD skin test for TB
- Blood test for illicit drugs
- Pregnancy test
- Endoscopic examination of nose and throat

If you elected to have the sputum sample analyzed in the microbiology lab you might have gotten a report back saying that they found "Acid-Fast Bacilli smear and culture positive" and those results strongly suggest that Manjula has TB or

Medical Investigation 101

Mycobacterium tuberculosis (also simply called tuberculosis) that she picked up during her trip to India.

You could easily spend months reading and learning about tuberculosis because this disease has such an extensive and long history. See if you can research which of these statements are true?

True or False:

- Tuberculosis still kills over a million people every year.
- About 2 out of 3 people test positive by a skin test (called a PPD or a Mantoux test) for TB exposure around the world.
- Although TB can attack many sites in the body, 90% of cases involve the lungs.
- TB resistant to the standard antibiotics that once cured TB has become a current world health crisis.

Additional thoughts about TB and insights:

Robert Heinrich Herman Koch (1843-1910) received the Nobel Prize in Physiology/Medicine for his remarkable research that allowed physicians to understand and treat TB. Koch was the first to think formally about how one would actually go about proving definitively what causes a disease. Suppose, for example, half of your class members at school become sick at their stomach tomorrow, and you suspect that they got sick from a contaminate in a treat someone brought into school for everyone to enjoy at a class celebration. How could you prove that the treat caused the illness? Koch said you would need to satisfy 4 conditions:

1. You would need to find the contaminant in everyone who got sick, but no contaminant in the students who did not get sick. But you cannot stop there.
2. The contaminant must be isolated from a sick student.
3. The isolated contaminant must then be able to make a healthy student sick.
4. The contaminant must then be isolated again from that healthy student now sick and shown to be identical to the original contaminant. (Koch was very thorough.)

Koch's postulates remain today as the established criteria for medical scientists to accept that a specific organism or substance actually constitute the true cause of a disease. You will recognize that Koch's postulates might actually serve as sound guidance, with some adjustments, for proving conclusions in many other areas of life and science. When two things seem to happen together the coincidence encourages us all to suspect that one thing caused the other. Koch's rules try to separate coincidence from causation, and not allow us to jump to the conclusion one thing caused the other. Only people with automobiles get into automobile accidents, so would you agree that cars cause accidents?

Mycobacterium tuberculosis has made people sick and die probably for just about as long as there were people on this earth. But now we have tuberculosis germs that no longer go away when treated with the antibiotic medications that almost always cured TB in the past. We believe that the germs evolve **resistance** to our drugs over time. You probably have a familiarity with the notion of **evolution**. We believe that genetic material, the RNA or DNA that makes possible living cells that can do many amazing things to include becoming human beings, can change over time to make living organisms better adapted to survive threats in their environment. We do not believe that process comes about from any actual intention or design, but rather from an accident. Not an automobile accident this time, but a mistake in the process of copying the genetic code inside cells. We think an accident or a mistake results in a new gene or combination of genes that makes a particular living organism better, and because of that new feature the new organism reproduces more successfully to make that feature become the new standard for that type of organism over many generations. If the accident makes the organism less advantaged in dealing with enemies or weaker in some other way, the trait fades away in future generations.

Why then would the Mycobacterium tuberculosis evolve to continue to cause disease in humans instead of human beings evolve to become resistant to the tubercular bacillus? Certainly, by acts of intention humans have come up with medications to fight off TB, and yet this tiny Mycobacterium seemingly "outsmarts" those medications invented by scientists. The answer lies in what we said about evolution; the accidental improvements in the living species take generations to become the norm. A generation for humans occurs in the order to 20 years. A generation for a Mycobacterium occurs about every 18 hours, actually a long generation time compared to many bacteria that divide more than twice an hour. For every generation of humans, Mycobacteria have nearly 10,000 generations. That difference in generation duration represents a huge biological advantage for the evolution of microscopic organisms. Thank goodness lions, tigers, and snakes have generations much more closely aligned with our own!

You live in an era in which molecular biology continually unlocks the secrets of the genes, how they work and what they can do. As a consequence, you might very reasonably expect that in the not too distant future someone might figure out how to manipulate a virus that selectively makes the Mycobacterium tuberculosis sick. That virus might save millions of human lives and that sort of new genetic biology thinking appears increasingly popular in the fight not only against infections, but also against cancer.

And while you are thinking about the mechanism of evolution, have you ever thought about how your favorite flower evolved such a lovely **visage**? Again, we do not believe the design came about due to any intention on the part of the plant; instead, the beauty of the flower represents an accidental advantage the plant has in regard to its environment. The plant has no eyes with which to even evaluate its beauty. What eyes do see the flower and turn its beauty into an advantage?

Investigation 3.8B: Respiratory System

Tuberculosis is a contagious disease that affects mainly the lungs, the key organ of the **respiratory system**. Our lungs exchange the waste product of metabolism (burning food for energy) **carbon dioxide** for life-sustaining **oxygen** that we also need for deriving energy from the food we eat.

Humans, indeed all primates, have two lungs. Your lungs are located in your chest, or **thorax**. They are connected to the atmosphere by way of the **trachea**, which ends at the **epiglottis**. Your epiglottis is a protective cover designed to keep food from entering your trachea. The trachea receives air from the mouth and nose. Go ahead, cover your nostrils and breathe in through your mouth. Now close your mouth and breathe in through only your nose. You should still be conscious and feeling well; breathing through either your nose or mouth results in air passing to your lungs.

Sometimes we can only breathe through our mouth; think about the last time you had a stuffy nose and could barely breathe at all through your nose. You definitely did some mouth breathing then. What happens when you are eating a meal and your parent reminds you to keep your mouth closed while chewing? In that case you would probably need to do your breathing through your nose.

Air (21% oxygen, 78% nitrogen, and the rest water vapor, carbon dioxide, and rare gases) enters the trachea from either your mouth or nose and is pushed down into the lung bronchi by atmospheric pressure as your muscles expand the volume of your chest cavity. Are you asking yourself what happens to the other stuff in the air that is not oxygen? That's an excellent question. We think mainly of oxygen passing through the lung tissue into our blood stream and carbon dioxide coming out. Nitrogen and other gases also pass through but because they do not participate in the body's chemical processes they are said to come to equilibrium, which means as many molecules wander in as wander out. So, under normal conditions it appears as if nitrogen does not pass through the lungs at all. If you should read about deep sea diving you will learn that nitrogen has in fact passed into the body and can become quite important to divers who come to the surface too quickly after diving to great depths.

Dust and other pollutants that might float about in the air we breathe we hope get filtered from the air on its way down the trachea and bronchi by hair-like villi covered in sticky mucus lining the surface. If you have ever blown your nose on a white tissue after being in a very dust place, you may have seen the evidence of this filtering process.

Cigarette smokers over time destroy the protective villi and disrupt their amazing ability to move that sticky mucus up and out of the trachea. Continued smoking can keep the trachea and bronchi irritated resulting in the cough characteristic of chronic bronchitis (a word meaning inflammation of the bronchi).

The bronchi break into smaller units called bronchioles until the air finally reaches the microscopic air sacs called alveoli. Air is passed from the alveoli into the capillaries and carbon dioxide, a waste product of your body metabolism, passes from the capillaries to the alveoli, where it passes from the alveoli to bronchioles to bronchi, then up the trachea and is exhaled by the mouth or nose.

Medical Investigation 101

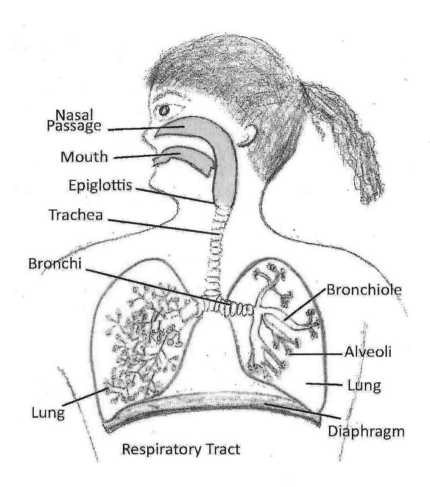

The lungs are covered on the outside by a thin lining called the pleura. The pleura also lines the inside of the chest cavity. The pleural membranes excrete a lubricant. If they weren't lubricated the pleural membranes would not slide smoothly to allow the lung to expand when you take a breath by tightening muscles that expand the chest cavity. Your right lung has three lobes while the left has two. Perhaps the left lung has one less lobe to make room for your heart.

The process of air inhalation followed by exhalation we call breathing or **respiration**. Respiration is an active, not passive process. Inspiration (drawing in air) is an active process resulting from contraction of your intercostal muscles and diaphragm. The **diaphragm** is a very strong muscle separating your chest from your abdomen. Exhalation can be a passive, powered by the elasticity of our lung pushing the air out so it can contract to its relaxed volume. You don't have to use any muscles at all for exhalation. You probably also recognize that you can switch exhalation into an active process when you want to blow out the candles on a birthday cake.

Because our lungs are processing air from our external environment, toxins and infectious microbes, both living and non-living can find their way into our lungs. When that happens, we rely on our immune system to fight back and keep us healthy. That plan has been known to fail from time to time.

Toxic chemicals in the air can enter our lungs and cause damage. Many people suffer from chronic diseases caused by long-term exposure to chemicals found in urban communities or perhaps at their work site. Governments and private organizations work to identify and remove these health threats and it makes sense for us all to support these efforts.

Almost everyone who smokes for many years will end up with some degree of **emphysema**. This disease results in damage to the alveoli and a loss of elasticity in the lung tissue itself. These changes make it difficult to move air in and out, and also to get oxygen into the blood stream. Emphysema patients are sometimes called "pink puffers" or "blue blotters" depending upon which problem in breathing dominates. If the parents coming to your medical office smoke in your presence, please ask them to refrain, for your health can be affected as well. Smokers also have an increased risk of lung cancer because of a **carcinogenic** chemical found in cigarette smoke.

In addition to the toxic chemicals attacking our lungs from our environment, our lungs are exposed to disease-causing microbes. There are hundreds of such infectious diseases capable of airborne spread.

Tuberculosis, as we learned in this case history, is a bacterial infection contracted by breathing in organisms from the air from infected people. How can you avoid breathing? Obviously, you can't. It is particularly disturbing when you realize that airborne pathogens can stay in the air after the infected person

Medical Investigation 101

has left the room. You may have no knowledge of your exposure to these pathogens whatsoever. The best defense is a healthy immune system. Just because you are exposed to an airborne pathogen does not mean you will definitely get sick. More often than we probably realize our immune system recognizes the bad guys you inhale and attacks and conquers them before they can establish themselves within our respiratory system.

We rely constantly on our respiratory system to provide us breathable air and filter out dirt, pollen, and pollutants. Our respiratory system works very well most of the time with our immune system working to keep us healthy. It's important to keep our lungs healthy by not smoking and avoiding smog, dust, and toxic vapors as best we can.

Investigation 3.9

3.9A: Abdominal Pain & Dark Urine
3.9B: Urinary Tract

Investigation 3.9A: Abdominal Pain and Dark Urine

Introduction:

Who are you? We are not looking to learn your name. We are conducting investigations in this book to find the causes of various medical **symptoms** in order to better understand medical science, and in the process see if you might consider selecting some particular area of healthcare as your career. But in this investigation, you will first need to figure out the name of the healthcare role you are playing. You have frequently played the role of a primary care physician, but not today.

You start this morning, not in a doctor's office, but at the hospital. You came in from the physician's parking lot through a security door with an electronic combination that required you to press 1-8-4-6-#, a security number selected by the medical staff to honor the year of the first public demonstration of **general anesthesia**. General anesthesia constitutes America's greatest contribution to healthcare. Dentist William Thomas Green Morton conducted that demonstration of general anesthesia at the Massachusetts General Hospital in Boston on October 16, 1846. Now we find it difficult to imagine what people were forced to endure prior to 1846. The ability to do general anesthesia and make people **unconscious** for painful procedures came along only relatively recently in the long history of medicine. In any case, you plugged-in the right numbers and successfully opened the back door of the hospital.

As you head toward the in-patient section of the hospital you pass by the entrance to the Operating Rooms, but you keep going straight ahead. When you first got interested in medicine you were fascinated by the puzzle of the **medical diagnosis**, but you worried that you might not be able to handle the "blood and gore" of medical care. You later discovered that everyone who considers a **career** in healthcare had that same concern. Will I faint when I really need to take action? In truth, once you get **immersed** into medical training and actually come face-to-face with some **gory** situations, to your surprise, you barely notice. Instead you have so much to think about and remember as you start doing what needs to be done, your mind never even registers that gore. Gore bothers spectators, not healthcare providers. If you feel healthcare calling you,

you need not worry for a moment about how you would handle "blood and gore." But in your role today, you will never step foot into the **operating room** or see anything **grotesque**.

You are on your way to see a patient at the request of a **colleague** in **internal medicine**. Today you play the role of a **medical consultant**. Your internist colleague, Dr. Brian Johnson, has admitted a 38-year-old female to the hospital and wants your help in sorting through her problems and suggesting the right treatment. You start your **consultation** by reading Dr. Johnson's History and Physical in the patient's **hospital chart**. (Remember you are still trying to identify the consulting role you play today.)

Chief Complaint:

"My urine has looked red, off and on, for about a week, and for the last two days I have had pains in my stomach and lower back, really severe last night."

History of Present Illness:

Martha Benson came into my practice about 8 years ago. I have seen her for annual physical examinations and routine care for minor infections, lumps and bumps, weight control, and **immunizations**, but nothing significant except a steady trend toward **hypertension**. I finally put her on a blood pressure medication two years ago, but I am not satisfied that I have adequately controlled her blood pressure. Now she has pain, **hematuria**, loss of appetite, and symptoms suggesting significant **kidney** issues. In the office we found 4+ hematuria, no evidence of a **kidney infection**, no history of trauma, and I am concerned. I elected to bring her into the hospital to get to the bottom of this quickly and to deal with her pain.

Review of Systems:

She had both measles and chicken pox as a child. Her parents made sure she got her childhood immunizations and she gets flu shots annually. She has had no surgery ever and came to the hospital only for an uneventful delivery of a healthy daughter 9 years ago. She has had no problems ever with her heart,

Medical Investigation 101

lungs, kidneys, stomach, or nervous system, but I see in my office notes that I have treated her twice for **urinary tract** infections, both cleared uneventfully.

Medications: Lisinopril 10 mg once daily
Allergies: none

Examination:

Wt: 135 lbs.   Respirations: 18 /min   Pulse: 84 /min
Blood Pressure: 148/94   Temperature: 98.2° F.
General: Healthy appearing young female, well developed, well nourished, with abdominal pain.
Head: No abnormal findings. No enlarged lymph nodes. No redness in the ears or throat. Normal range of movement of the neck. No thyroid enlargement.
Heart: No abnormal sounds
Lungs: Clear
Abdomen: Normal bowel sounds. Abdominal tenderness present, mainly in her **flanks**. **Percussion** of her lower back produces significant discomfort.
Extremities: No deformities. No swelling. No tenderness.
Neurologic: Grossly intact.

Assessment: Normally healthy and active young woman, mother, uncomfortable and concerned. I consider new onset hematuria along with hypertension at a relatively young age not easily controlled to warrant thorough evaluation and I have asked for a consultation to help sort this out.

Dr. Johnson has asked **you** to figure out Martha's problem. What type of physician will you call yourself when you introduce yourself to your new patient? (Select from one of the following)

- Obstetrician
- Nephrologist
- Urologist
- Gastroenterologist

Before you see the patient make sure you find out what hematuria means. Did you look it up?

And what sort of medication is Lisinopril?

If you search for a **differential diagnosis** for Martha's symptoms you will generate a very long list that contains problems with many organs other than the **kidneys**. Dr. Johnson has focused on the kidney and has asked for help with the kidney in mind, but as a consultant you know better than to dismiss the possibility of other organ issues. But you agree it makes sense to focus first on the kidney.

Is there anything in the history or not in the history that makes you agree with Dr. Johnson's belief that the kidney demands your primary attention?

Nephrologists and **urologists** often say they got interested in the kidney because they have ready access to the chemistry of what goes in and what comes out. The blood flows into and through the kidney and urine comes out. The kidneys clean waste products out of the bloodstream and regulate the levels of certain chemicals that we need in our blood. The design of the kidney normally keeps all the red blood cells inside the blood vessels that feed blood into and out of the organ. When blood cells show up in significant numbers in the urine, enough to make the urine red, the patient needs an accurate diagnosis. Martha should not have red blood cells in her urine.

We credit a physician named Mark Ravitch with an often-repeated quotation, "The dumbest kidney is smarter than the smartest doctor." Ravitch was drawing attention to the amazing ability of the kidney to separate out the fluid portion of the blood from the red blood cells and then to selectively put back into the bloodstream only the molecules the body needs, allowing the others to become eliminated from the body in urine. Furthermore, it appears the kidney does the right thing, sometimes despite the efforts of a well-meaning but mistaken physician. The kidney has a complex function, and its cells carry out complex chemistry and physiology, so when something goes wrong the problem readily deserves a specialist to find the cause. Indeed, the kidney does appear to deserve Dr. Ravitch's compliment.

Medical Investigation 101

As a consulting physician focused on the kidney you have a differential diagnosis list of kidney-based diseases you especially want to rule out quickly for Dr. Johnson and Martha. The problem could lie outside the kidney, but if that proves the case Dr. Johnson may need a different consultant.

Your Focused Differential Diagnosis List:

- **Urinary Infection**
- **Pylonephritis**
- **Kidney Stone**
- **Upper Urinary Tract Obstruction**
- **Cystitis**
- **Kidney Cancer**
- **Polycystic Kidney Disease**
- **Leptospirosis**

The following chart will provide a little more information about the symptoms of each disease on the differential diagnosis list:

Disease	Nausea/ Vomit	Pain	Pain	Painful Urination	Fever/ Chills	Hematuria	Frequent Urination	Other
Urinary Infection	X	Upper back	side	X	X	X	X	acute
Pyelo-nephritis	X	Upper back	side	X	X		X	Acute or chronic
Kidney Stones	X	Sudden, severe abdominal				X		acute
Upper Urinary Tract Infection	X		side	X	X		X	acute
Cystitis		pelvic		X	X	X	X	Acute or chronic
Kidney Cancer		Low back or none	mass		X	X		Appetite loss
Polycystic Kidney Disease		abdominal	Low Back sides	If kidney stones		X	X	Hyper-tension chronic
Leptso-spirosis	X	Headache, low back,	calf		X			Jaundice, appetite loss

After asking the nurse on duty in which room Martha can be found, you walk into her room to find her lying in her hospital bed. After introducing yourself to Martha, you then confirm the medical history from the chart with her before repeating most of the examination that Dr. Johnson did previously. You double-check Dr. Johnson for two reasons. First you might find something that Dr. Johnson missed, and second, you might find something has changed since Dr. Johnson examined the patient. Consulting physicians often find a clue the primary physician lacked simply because they get to the patient later in the process of the illness. In Martha's case you did not find any new information.

On admission to the hospital Dr. Johnson had ordered **blood chemistry** studies on Martha that included measuring the levels of **blood urea nitrogen** and **creatinine.** These tests measure the amount of waste products still in the blood that the kidney should have removed. The lab calculated an estimate of Martha's **kidney filtration rate** (estimated GFR) of 64 mL/minute, when a normal value should exceed 90. You see that Martha's kidneys are not working properly and you decide to ask for help from the department of **radiology** to figure out precisely what is happening. You may have heard the expression, "A picture is worth a thousand words."

An X-ray picture of the kidney called an **intravenous pyelogram** (IVP) uses an **iodinated** contrast material **injected** into a **vein** to make the blood and then the urine visible. The X-ray pictures taken over a period of time after the injection tell us what is happening in the kidney and the ureters that take the urine down to the **urinary bladder**. While you would love to have that information, the fact that Martha's kidneys are not working efficiently causes you to reconsider. The contrast material can often injure a kidney so the IVP might possibly make Martha's condition worse. So, you decide to ask the radiologist to image Martha's kidneys not with X-rays but with **ultrasound** (sound waves much higher in frequency than our ears can hear).

You have several other patients to see in the hospital, so two hours later you walk to the radiology department to review the ultrasound study with the **radiologist**. The study demonstrates five **kidney cysts**, two in the left kidney and three in the right. Those findings confirm the diagnosis of **Autosomal Dominant** Polycystic Kidney Disease, a condition that we do not know how to cure, but a condition that healthcare providers can work with patients to manage.

Polycystic Kidney Disease does cause blood pressure problems because the kidneys play a key role in **regulation** of blood pressure. Dr. Johnson actually has Martha on the right blood pressure medicine, but he will need to continue to work on controlling her blood pressure.

Polycystic Kidney Disease can also create cysts in other parts of the body, abnormalities in blood vessels in the brain, and even leaking in the valves of the heart, all issues Dr. Johnson will have to watch for in Martha. Urinary tract infections appear more commonly in patients with this disorder.

As a consultant you immediately get in touch with Dr. Johnson to discuss your diagnosis. Dr. Johnson may wish to explain the situation with his patient himself and he may want you to also follow Martha in the future. You ask Dr. Johnson for permission to speak with Martha's daughter's pediatrician about the findings. Why would you make that request?

Would Martha ever be a candidate for a kidney transplant?

If you still have curiosity about how the kidney does its "magic," you might look up the role it plays in regulating blood pressure and see if you can understand why Dr. Johnson was using the right blood pressure for Martha by looking up the mechanism of action for the medication Lisinopril.

Polycystic kidney disease will change Martha's life. She did not do anything to cause this disease. No one wants the job of sitting down with Martha to tell her the results of her ultrasound examination. No one wants to tell her that we do not know how to cure her condition. Delivering bad news, unfortunately, remains a task that falls on healthcare professionals to perform.

One of the important skills in the practice of medicine we call the "**bedside manner.**" While our lessons here have focused on the path to finding the right diagnosis, you can certainly appreciate also that medicine involves difficult conversations all too often. Patients want the professionals who take responsibility for their medical care to care not just about their body, but also to care genuinely for them as individuals with hopes and fears and failings and passions. Fortunately, the ability to learn and use science does not **preclude** the ability to also relate to others with compassion and understanding.

Investigation 3.9B: Urinary Tract

The **kidneys** are part of the **urinary tract**, which is responsible for eliminating liquid waste and extra water filtered from our blood, without expelling the blood's red and white cells and platelets. Waste products are like trash; you take out the trash so it doesn't accumulate. The same is true for your body. The process of eliminating or retaining fluid waste also affects our **blood pressure**. Consider this: If your vascular system retains too much fluid it places an extra work load on the heart; your heart tries to pump everything that the veins return. If you have too little fluid retained in your blood vessels your blood pressure drops, reducing the blood flow to vital organs. In this case you might feel weak, perhaps even faint when you arise quickly to go play outside. To maintain the right amount of blood volume and blood pressure inside vessels the kidneys make a **hormone** that can **constrict** the **arteries**, keeping blood pressure from getting too low while the kidneys start returning water and salts filtered from the blood stream back into the veins that then leave the kidneys. So, the kidneys regulate the volume of the vascular system and also the **resistance** to the flow of the blood which causes the blood pressure in arteries to climb upward.

The urinary tract includes your kidneys, **ureters**, **bladder**, and **urethra**.

Kidneys

In the medical world "**renal**" refers to anything related to the kidneys. **Renal failure** means the kidneys have stopped working. A **Renal biopsy** is a sample of kidney tissue. The kidneys get their blood supply from the **renal artery**. Blood leaves the kidneys through the **renal veins**. Renal disease is a sickness related to the kidneys. Most people are born with two kidneys. Sometimes a generous person will donate one kidney to someone whose kidneys have both failed. Such a donation gives the recipient a second chance at a normal life.

Once inside the kidney, the blood goes through a filtering process to remove waste products collected as the blood moves throughout the body. It works a little like a coffee filter, which prevents coffee grounds from slipping through to the coffee cup. The kidneys filter the blood so that all the blood cells, plus some of the large protein molecules like albumen, stay inside blood vessels and leave the kidneys, less the waste products brought in by the arteries. Then the **nephrons** (tiny tubes lined with very clever cells that do the kidney's job) go to work on the fluid portion separated from the bloodstream and pull out sugar, salt, potassium, a few other molecules, plus water if needed, and put those useful substances back into the bloodstream in the concentrations the rest of our body likes to see. Each day an adult's two kidneys filter about 150 quarts of fluid (called **filtrate**) out of the bloodstream, returning components we can still use back into the blood, and produces one to two quarts of urine depending upon how many beverages the individual enjoyed that day. Each kidney has around a million nephrons that do this complex filtering that eliminates waste but preserves the chemicals our body still needs. More than 99% of everything passing through the nephrons can return to the renal vein and go back into our circulation, especially if you are walking across a desert with no canteen of water. An infection in the nephrons can affect the kidney's ability to do this complex chemical sorting task. You can help keep your kidneys filtering efficiently by drinking six to eight glasses of water each day to keep your nephrons from getting clogged up with waste! On a very hot day when you are exercising, your body loses salts in sweat, so you might elect to drink a sports drink to replace those salts and help your kidneys keep everything in balance.

The collected waste filtered by the nephrons is urine, or pee. It drips into a tube connected at the other end to the **urinary bladder**. What makes pee go to the bladder? Gravity, of course. The kidneys are located at the level of the middle of your back on both sides while the bladder is located well below your belly button. Gravity makes the urine flow downhill to the bladder. What allows urine to travel to the bladder while you sleep, you ask? The ureter has smooth muscle cells in its walls that squeeze in a coordinated way to keep the pee moving in the right direction, even while you sleep (even if you sleep head down hanging from a trapeze... but don't try that).

Urine is constantly under production, yet thankfully we don't have to go pee all the time. We have a special place to store urine until we find a convenient time to visit a bathroom. The bladder is our urine storage tank. Our bladder enlarges like a balloon as it fills with urine; it also contracts in size as it empties during urination. Typically, our bladder is about two inches in diameter, but has the ability to enlarge if needed to six inches in length, when we can't find a bathroom. We have stretch sensors in the bladder wall that tell us when we need to pee; this is known as the **micturition reflex**. Our bladder has a **sphincter** that acts like a faucet; it opens to let urine out and closes to stop the flow. Sometimes due to illness or injury patients partially lose control of their bladder sphincter and suffer leakage. Pampers for adults can treat this problem. Those who lose total bladder control can wear a **urinary catheter** and **urine bag**, which collects their urine outside of their body. Everyone must eliminate waste products one way or another. One might expect such a simple structure as the urethra would never create a reason to consult a physician. Nope! One of the most common medical problems effecting males beyond the age of 65 years-old arises from external pressure on the urethra caused by gradual enlargement of the prostate gland. Fortunately, a recently developed office procedure may soon give urologists a powerful tool to quickly correct that condition.

When **urine** is released by relaxation of the bladder sphincter it is still inside our body. In order to reach the outside world urine must travel through the **urethra**, the final leg of the journey. The trip is longer for boys than girls, the shorter distance putting girls at greater risk of bacterial infections in that area. Sometimes the urethra becomes too narrow to allow a smooth flow of urine; this can make peeing a slow and sometimes painful process.

Here is a look at the system that gets that done for you.

Urinary Tract

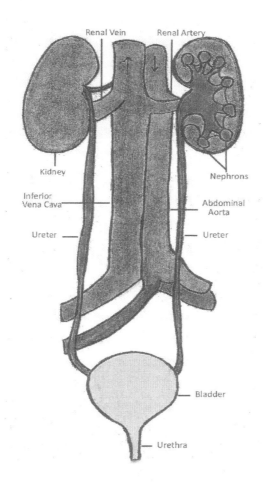

We cannot live without eliminating waste from our bloodstream. Our urinary tract constantly produces urine that we eliminate when we get the urge. Medical textbooks have long taught that urine coming from the kidney contains no bacteria. Recent research has found that urine itself is not **sterile** as it exits

Medical Investigation 101

your body but contains small amounts of bacteria that normally reside in the wall of the bladder. Significant amounts of bacteria in the urine still suggest an infection. Our urine is about 95% water, but also contains significant amounts of nitrogen containing compounds plus chloride, potassium, and other compounds. Where did all that **nitrogen** come from? What is the major component of the air we breathe in? Nitrogen, of course! However, the nitrogen in our urine did not come from our lungs, but from our stomach. Urine nitrogen enters our bloodstream as a byproduct of the metabolism of dietary protein components inside cells, protein components that allow our body grow and to repair itself.

Investigation 3.10

3.10A: Weak & Dizzy
3.10B: Environmental Toxins

Investigation 3.10A: Weak and Dizzy

Introduction:

When medical students start seeing actual patients under the supervision of resident and faculty physicians, they quickly learn to dread the patient whose Chief Complaint reads, "I feel weak and dizzy." Such a chief complaint occurs frequently. The dread comes from the lack of **specificity**. The **differential diagnosis** of weak and dizzy could include hundreds of conditions, while a routine examination with lab work often may find nothing abnormal.

Guess what! This morning your first patient in your office appears on your schedule as "Dorothy Westfield, 78-year-old female, new patient, feeling weak and dizzy last few days. Brenda Kravetz, her daughter, scheduled the appointment.

Still feeling that old sense of dread, you head for Exam Room 3, remembering Brenda as a patient you have had in your practice for years. Brenda has two sons, both were attending college, but perhaps the oldest may now have graduated.

Chief Complaint and History of Present Illness:

You greet Brenda and introduce yourself to her Mother. Brenda explains that her retired Father's doctor in Chicago had found that her Father had advanced pancreatic cancer five months ago. Her Father fought hard but died six weeks ago. Mrs. Westfield, his widow, had agreed to come live with her daughter Brenda while they sorted out the **estate**. Brenda and her husband were thinking they might just add a room onto their house and keep Dorothy with them indefinitely. But, over the last few days Dorothy Westfield, who had navigated the last five difficult months valiantly, seemed no longer her previously vigorous self. Now she has no interest in going anywhere except back to bed. She is not stable on her feet. She complains of aches in her feet and hands. Her appetite has waned and Brenda added that her Mother has complained of stomach discomfort and diarrhea.

Physical Examination

The nurse has left you Dorothy's vital signs on the front of a new chart:
Weight: 132   BP: 127/73   Pulse: 94   Respirations: 24   Temp: 98.8 F.

Dorothy Westfield appears sick, although her body looks well developed suggesting no long history of illness. But today she definitely seems **listless** and **disengaged**. She answers direct questions but has no interest in a conversation. You find no abnormalities of the head and neck, except her mouth seems very dry. No enlarged **lymph nodes**. Her heart and lungs sound normal. **Palpation** of the abdomen evokes some reaction of discomfort, not severe but definitely real. The **liver** does not seem enlarged. Dorothy's skin appears dry. Her hands and feet appear normal although you do see a little swelling of the feet and ankles. You find some scattered areas of **hyperpigmentation** of the skin, but such findings are common in persons of her age.

Medical History

Dorothy's daughter, Brenda, answers most of your questions addressed to her Mother. Dorothy has led an active life, working originally as a high school English teacher, who also coached a very successful debate team. She married and raised two healthy children and filled her time after the children left home with oil painting and directing plays at a community theatre. She had no major surgery and took no medications, except for vitamins and some oral and topical **estrogen** replacements. She has had age appropriate **vaccines** for prevention of **pneumonia** and **shingles**, and periodic **tetanus boosters**. She has not traveled outside the country in the previous year.

Make a mental list of Dorothy Westfield's signs and symptoms that you would use to create a differential diagnosis. Do you appreciate the dread of the "weak and dizzy" complaint? Nothing jumps out, but you feel confident of something abnormal that you need to track down.

The "Isabel" differential diagnosis software provides you with the following list of possible causes for Dorothy's symptoms: **Diabetic Neuropathy, Pernicious Anemia, Addison's Disease, Vitamin B12 Deficiency, Pancreatic Cancer, Brucellosis, Celiac Disease, Heavy Metal Intoxication, Pancreatitis, Cirrhosis, Compartment Syndrome, Food Poisoning, Iron Deficiency Anemia, Crohn's Disease, Hepatitis A, Endocarditis, Rheumatoid Arthritis, Malignant Atrophic Papulosis, Transient Ischemic Attack, Polyneuropathy Disorder, and Postural Orthostatic Tachycardia Syndrome.**

The list jumps all over the body, even to include Pancreatic Cancer, which caused Dorothy's husband's death. Where do you even start?

Which lab tests would you order to begin the process? This choice we expect to prove very difficult. You want to find a clue to the problem, but not spend thousands of dollars testing everything at once unless you think the patient has a condition that threatens her life over the next few days. Try to select a few simple tests that might point you in the right direction. You can then elect other tests down the road to get the right diagnosis.

- Combined Blood Count (CBC) to check for anemia and B12 deficiency.
- Electrolytes and Blood Urea Nitrogen to check on kidney function.
- Chest X-ray
- Heavy Metals Panel, blood test to check for arsenic, mercury, and lead.
- Complete blood metabolic panel to evaluate for liver function.
- Cardiac enzymes to rule out a heart attack.

- Blood culture to look for infection in the blood stream.
- Electromyogram (EMG) to measure conduction velocity in nerves.
- Cardiac angiography to evaluate circulation of blood to the heart.
- Acute Hepatitis Panel to rule out Hepatitis A, B, or C.
- Antinuclear Antibody (ANA) and Rheumatoid Factor blood test.
- Halter Monitor for detection of episodes of tachycardia
- Urinalysis
- X-rays of hands and feet.

In your office you can do a quick test for severe anemia and also get an idea of dehydration, so you elect to do that before anything else. If you selected other tests, they will require the hospital labs and those results will not be available until tomorrow at the earliest. Your nurse tells you in just a few minutes that Dorothy does not have a significant anemia but clearly needs some fluid replacement, perhaps because of the diarrhea she reported having which would drain water from her body.

You sit down with Dorothy and her daughter and explain what you have learned, and more importantly, what you still need to figure out. You will get all the results from the hospital laboratory back the next day, and you want to see Dorothy back in your office in 48 hours. In the meantime, you ask Brenda to insist that her mother drink Gatorade® and eat as best she can. If she cannot eat regular meals she should try to get down a nutrition drink like Ensure® or Boost®. And obviously, if anything changes, call your office day or night.

Now, fast forward 48 hours. Dorothy and Brenda have returned to your office. Brenda reports not much has changed. Dorothy has tried to eat and drink fluids. She has continued to have all of her symptoms reported before, remains weak and listless, still has aches, still has diarrhea, and vomited once after working hard to drink a glass of Boost®. You report that the lab tests you ran confirm a systemic illness that appears to affect Dorothy's liver and kidneys, producing mild impairment. Today you want to figure out the next step to getting to the root cause.

What would you do next? Before you read further, jot down your best idea for the next step. Perhaps you want to do an additional lab test from the list you considered before. Perhaps you want to ask a question not previously asked. This case does not seem to have any simple solution. Think about what you might do next?

Thank you for thinking hard about what you might do next for Dorothy. Practicing physicians in this same situation might indeed order more testing. They might also think of getting help from a specialist. It would not be unusual for a primary care physician faced with this case you are struggling to solve to send Dorothy to a Gastroenterologist since the most **definitive** symptoms appear to involve the stomach, intestines, and liver. But if you happened to write in the blank space above a different approach, especially if you would examine the patient again very thoroughly; please consider yourself exceptionally talented in medical science. You came up with the very best answer.

Today as you repeat your physical examination of Dorothy Westfield you discover three new findings. First, you detect some yellowing of the normally white surface of Dorothy's eye, a condition called **conjunctival** or **scleral icterus**. That finding points you toward disease in the liver, or hepatitis. Next you seek to feel or **palpate** the liver's edge under Dorothy's rib cage and find it easily since it sticks out significantly below the rib. Touching it proves uncomfortable for Dorothy. This confirms a liver issue in your mind. Next you look carefully at Dorothy's hands and you find a distinct white line stretching across the base of her finger nails, a mark that was not visible there 48 hours earlier. Most physicians would need to refresh their memory using a textbook to recall the name of such lines. The textbook calls them **Mees' lines** or **leukonychia striata** (leuko = white; nychia = nail; striata = lines). Medicine sure has a lot of big words.

The textbook also says that these Mees' lines appear when a patient has been poisoned with heavy metals, especially **arsenic**. Now you are ready to order that **Heavy Metals Panel** from the list you reviewed earlier. (Did you decide to do that test before, or did we talk you out of it?)

Now that you have gotten to this point in your study of medical science, you are thinking like a physician. You have a patient before you who displays symptoms you believe come from **chronic arsenic poisoning**. The treatment she needs now involves a process of chemically **binding** the arsenic so that she can eliminate it from her body in her urine. Physicians call this treatment **chelating** and it involves the **intravenous infusion** of a chelating agent like Dimercaprol. So while Dorothy needs to go to the hospital for a Heavy Metals Panel followed by treatment, you need to think about how all of this came about.

Arsenic has a very long and interesting history as an **instrument** of murder because, as you have seen, one could blame the early symptoms on other causes. Arsenic has been used over the centuries to kill rats and insects, to preserve wood, to color paint, and even added to medicines in low doses. With that many uses, you can appreciate that our ancestors could have easily obtained arsenic whenever they might have the need. Before the twentieth century aboratory tests to identify the presence of arsenic proved difficult to carry out reliably, so many murderers probably were never discovered.

Arsenic poisoning appears to have a much wider array of symptoms than we have come to expect in our search for a diagnosis. Why? The answer lies in the mechanism by which arsenic affects the human body. This chemical disrupts very basic reactions that all cells have in common as they **extract** energy from food and use that energy to create complex molecules from simpler ones. The poison, therefore, causes malfunctioning in every organ in the body, so the symptoms appear everywhere in a very confusing fashion.

Has Brenda or someone else in the family been feeding Dorothy some arsenic? Had someone decided they would prefer her life ended soon? Is this a matter for the police? If the police were involved would Dorothy no longer have a place to live protected by people who love her? Certainly, at this moment you cannot tell Brenda what you think might be happening.

Many times, in life and in medical practice, one must decide on a single path of action among many possible paths, when all paths seem less than **optimal**. The authors of this book know of an actual case similar to Dorothy's in which a physician discovered chronic arsenic poisoning after struggling to understand his elderly patient's symptoms. Then he too struggled to decide what to do. Finally, he simply confronted all the members of the household, except the patient, as a group with his findings, promising to go to the police if any future blood test showed arsenic or anything else bizarre happened to his patient. The patient continued to live happily in that household without further incident. Was that the best solution for all concerned? You can judge for yourself. This case illustrates the diversity of situations one can encounter in the practice of medicine.

So, what is arsenic? Arsenic is chemical element number 33 on the periodic table. It occurs in nature as a **metalloid** in water, rocks and soil; it is also found in manmade products. It happens to be highly toxic to humans. Most ingested arsenic is eliminated from our body in a few days, however, arsenic can be detected in nails and hair for up to a year after exposure.

One of the problems with arsenic arises because it occurs naturally in well water, and even in the soil. As fruits and vegetables grow the arsenic in the water or soil is absorbed into the plant. One of the largest episodes of deadly poisoning ever described occurred in Bangladesh because of an arsenic contaminated water supply. Attempted murder is not the only means of incurring arsenic poisoning.

Even without the results of heavy metal testing we see that some of Dorothy's symptoms are consistent with those expected in arsenic toxicity. Test results would, of course, confirm our diagnosis.

Arsenic toxicity primarily affects our skin, lungs, bladder, liver, and kidneys. Looking at Dorothy's symptoms we see many signs related to these areas.

Dorothy's skin is dry, most likely from dehydration associated with not eating and with vomiting. She also had areas of hyperpigmentation, which could be caused by arsenic toxicity.

Most significant was the finding off Mees' lines in her fingernails noted in the second, more thorough examination. The skin and hair are extensions of the skin; Mee's lines are indicative of arsenic exposure at least five or more weeks.

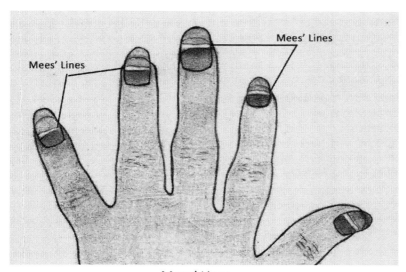

Mees' Lines

Testing of Dorothy's hair could provide further evidence of when exactly her arsenic exposure began.

Arsenic is **metabolized** in the liver. Chronic arsenic exposure experts believe can cause liver cancer. When Dorothy returned to the office her liver was enlarged and tender to palpation, suggesting arsenic was irritating and swelling her liver.

Arsenic is then **excreted** by the kidneys, causing damage demonstrated by the presence of blood in the urine; prolonged arsenic exposure causes cancer there as well.

The lungs are also damaged by arsenic exposure. What clue was present in Dorothy's vital signs that she might have early signs of **pulmonary** damage? Did you notice that her respiratory rate was 24 breaths per minute? That is a very non-specific finding, but it could be another clue to this unusual medical puzzle. Prolonged exposure to arsenic is thought to cause lung cancer.

Finally, arsenic is toxic to the sensitive tissues of our **bladder**. After passing through the kidneys, the next stop on the way out of the body is a visit to the bladder. Prolonged exposure to arsenic can result in cancer of the bladder.

Surely you can see that arsenic is not a chemical we voluntarily ingest, but one that too often makes its way into our body without our knowledge. To protect people from arsenic, public health officials must test our community water supplies and make sure our fruits and vegetables are not grown in soil contaminated by arsenic. Fresh vegetables and fruits imported into the United States during the winter represent a special opportunity for arsenic toxicity. Potential danger can arise when we have scant knowledge of the water and soil conditions in the land that grows our food.

Investigation 3.10B: Environmental Toxins

Unfortunately, we live in a dangerous world, although we generally feel safe in our community. We understand that accidents occur, and sometimes criminals intentionally try to harm others. But we sometimes forget that potential dangers exist in our environment. You can literally become ill from the air you breathe. You can even become ill from the land over which you walk, the food you eat, or the water you drink right in your own home.

We tend to think that our living conditions are pretty good compared to those of people living in far away, relatively under-developed countries about which we read. But we have many of the same environment dangers here in the United States.

For the past several years an organization called *Pure Earth* has tracked environmental **toxins** around the world. They continue to rate lead as the number one most **debilitating** toxin in the entire world. You may have read about the health issues related to battery recycling plants in Mexico. Many U.S. companies apparently send their batteries to Mexico to reclaim the valuable metals that allow batteries to store energy. People processing these metals in Mexico do not enjoy the protections our government provides American workers, so Mexican workers more commonly face the dangers of chronic lead exposure.

Lead is a known neurotoxin; that means it attacks the **neurological** centers of the body. Children your age and younger are most susceptible to lead poisoning, which causes permanent brain and nerve damage. You may have heard about the problems of lead poisoning the children of Flint, Michigan; the lead in Flint, Michigan, did not come from the water. These children drank city water contaminated with lead **leaching** out of old pipes that carried water to their homes.

Lead was once a common ingredient in paint in our own country. Parents would paint their children's furniture pretty colors with lead-containing paint. Many babies suffered acute lead toxicity after chewing on the painted surfaces as they were teething.

Lead is used in the factories of heavy industry. It seeps into the air, soil, and water. The air can blow to areas where people live and breathe it in. Contaminated soil eventually moves the lead into the roots and leaves, so people can eat lead in lettuce, spinach, or other favorite vegetables. None of this is good for our environment. *Pure Earth* estimates 26 million people worldwide are at risk of the dangers of lead toxicity.

In our country and others, a variety of heavy metals contaminate the environment, to include cadmium, mercury, and arsenic.

Cadmium is a metal used in zinc mining, some fertilizers, batteries, and electroplating. When your parents order chrome rims for their car they encourage the use of cadmium. When the World Trade Center came down in the terror attack in 2001, one of the main toxins that affected the first responders was Cadmium used in the building itself. The trend toward battery powered cars, intended to reduce the use of fossil fuels, has increased the need for cadmium for batteries. Advances in technology often call for careful evaluations of the advantages weighed against the potential risks to human health and environmental safety.

Mercury is another heavy metal highly toxic to the human body. Years ago, all thermometers utilized mercury to measure our temperature to identity a fever. Other uses for mercury over past decades included electrical switches and appliances, florescent lights, barometers, and many other uses. Mercury was absorbed into the water and soil. It made its way to our lakes and oceans. Several species of fresh and salt-water fish contain high amounts of mercury, their consumption recommended only in limited amounts. These fish include many favorites, such as tuna, swordfish, shark, and King mackerel. Mercury is no longer used in fever thermometers; experts recommend alcohol or digital thermometers for taking the temperature of humans.

With increasing knowledge of the environmental hazards of heavy metals comes new concerns brought on by new technologies. Fracking may be an excellent example. This relatively new technology was designed to increase the production of natural gas. Later it was determined that poisonous chemicals were, in some cases, getting into the aquifers providing drinking water to entire communities.

Exposure to **radioactive** materials such as **radon** and **uranium** are considered a major concern in the United States and other countries involved in nuclear energy and weapons. When the authors of this book were your age the "Cold War" was in full swing; The Soviet Union versus the United States. We were always told that nuclear war was almost eminent. Many homes actually built underground shelters as an opportunity to hide out following total destruction by a nuclear bomb.

In search of more efficient electrical power, nuclear power plants were developed in America and other countries. **Nuclear power** plants bring inherent danger along with the promise of cheap energy. Russia suffered a nuclear disaster at its **Chernobyl** nuclear power plant in 1986. After all the years that have passed since that disaster, the area around the power plant remains uninhabitable today. You may recall the nuclear disaster that occurred in **Japan** in 2011 following the earthquake generated tsunami.

In addition to the dangers of radioactive nuclear material from bombs and power plants, natural radioactive material seep upward from within Earth. It is estimated that one in fifteen U.S. homes are exposed to excessive levels of **radon**.

Toxic radioactive materials are not such a risk in under developed countries; they don't have nuclear weapons nor nuclear power plants.

Exposure to some **plastics** affords a potential toxicity that may affect human health. PCB's (polychlorinated biphenyls), a type of plastic banned from use in America in 1976, spread before that year so far into our air, water, and soil that it remains in measurable concentrations today. Protracted exposure to PCB's may cause nerve damage and cancer of the brain or liver. Phthalates, another plastic used in shower curtains, furniture upholstery, and some toys, some experts have linked to human toxicity. Government agencies continue to study and minimize our exposure to chemicals that represent a threat to human health.

Pesticides represent another environmentally harmful agent. They represent something of a paradox, as their purpose is to eradicate another environmentally harmful agent: mosquitos and other pests. They are used mostly in agriculture to prevent crop destruction. Until 1972 **DDT** was the toxin of choice to eradicate insect pests until it was determined they caused cancer and neurological impairment in humans. By then they had contaminated our air, water, and soil so thoroughly that we still find traces of DDT in soil, water, and animal life today.

In addition to the environmental toxins introduced here, there are many more: materials such as asbestos used in construction, products still used today such as acetone and turpentine, and even discarded prescription drugs find their way into the air, soil and water. Inhaling nauseous fumes while painting your nails is not healthy. Human **prescriptions drugs** spreading in water have caused mutations in animals and fish and are even detectable in municipal water systems.

Since the beginning of the industrial age fossil fuels have provided the power that allows us to work and travel. For over one hundred years we have been burning fossil fuels and spewing huge amounts of carbon monoxide and dioxide into the air. As the world's population and industries grew while animals were replaced as the source of transportation by cars, trucks, buses, trains, and airplanes, our atmosphere filled up with the toxic gases produced. The result is a warming of our atmosphere and shift in the climate patterns on Earth.

Aside from changing climate, the quality of the air you and I breathe affects our health. The **World Health Organization** estimates the 4.6 million people die each year as a direct result of air pollution. Interestingly, most of the effects come from indoor chemical fume exposure. If you think about it, most people spend about 90% of their time indoors. We are bombarded by fumes coming from our carpets, stoves, heaters, fireplaces, and more. Even the walls of our homes can contain toxic chemicals that leech into the air where we breathe them into our unsuspecting lungs. Equally as harmful to our health, yet totally preventable, is the inhalation of **carcinogenic** chemical from **cigarette smoke**. Is it amazing to you that so many people continue to smoke when the dangers are posted right on the package? The companies practically tell the smoker they will get cancer yet smoking remains a pervasive problem. Unfortunately, many are exposed to cigarette toxins through second hand smoke.

At one time smoking was actually promoted as a healthy lifestyle by the **Surgeon General** of the United States. Of course, we now know that is totally untrue. Both of my parents smoked cigarettes when I was a child; I despised even the smell of smoke. I eventually made a deal with my parents: I would eat dinner with them if they wouldn't smoke at the table. I probably was otherwise unaware of the horrible smell of everything in our house, including our furniture and clothes. That would only be apparent to someone whose sense of smell had not accommodated to that odor. It is no wonder so many suffer from asthma and other respiratory diseases. **Chronic exposure** to these undetected toxins can cause cancer and other serious diseases.

We inhabit an environment loaded with potential to destroy our health and even end our life. As technology advances, along with the benefits, we seem to eventually find new hazards for concern. Is climate change really Earth's greatest problem? What do you think?

Investigation 3.11

3.11A: Foodborne Illness
3.11B: Case Study

Investigation 3.11A: Food-borne Illness

Although millions of people come down with foodborne illness each year, the average person rarely thinks about food safety when they get hungry. As a physician you will see many patients in your office with complaints of abdominal pain, nausea, vomiting, and diarrhea. Unfortunately, these symptoms are not specific to any particular disorder. Does your patient have the flu? Or might they suffer from a **food-borne illness**, commonly called **food poisoning**?

Food-borne illness is a common, yet costly **public health** issue, even in the United States. You might be surprised to learn that the CDC (**Centers for Disease Control and Prevention**) recognizes more than 250 different food-borne diseases; most are infections caused by a limited number of bacteria, viruses, and parasites. Would you believe one in six people come down with a food-borne illness each year? It is estimated that every year approximately 48 million people contract a food-borne illness; about 128,000 are hospitalized and 3,000 die. So, this is a serious problem!

As a physician you must rely on a good history and physical exam, plus a few special laboratory tests, to make the correct **diagnosis** in order to know how to treat this illness. Your patient's life could be in the balance. Even when you suspect food-borne illness, you need to identify the responsible organism to know how to treat. Your treatment plan depends on identifying the organism.

Food-borne illnesses can be divided into three major groups: **bacteria**, **viral**, and **parasitic**. Bacteria cause the most illness and the most common bacterial pathogens are **Salmonella**, Campylobacter, Listeria, Staphylococcus, and Clostridium Perfringens. There are fewer viruses and parasites responsible for food-borne illness, mainly Norovirus and, until recently, Hepatitis A. Parasites that cause disease in humans can also be **ingested** in food: Amoebiasis, Toxoplasmosis, and Trichinosis cause common parasitic illnesses.

Medical Investigation 101

Bacteria are microscopic, single-celled living organisms, some of which cause illness in humans. They live in soil, in water, even throughout the human body. Some need air to survive, some don't. Some are round-shaped, others are rod-shaped. Most grow best in a warm environment and grow slower or stop growing in a cool environment. Some make us sick, while others are necessary for our survival. Bacteria that make us ill we call **pathogens**.

Bacterial food-borne pathogens have several features in common, so we need to focus on their differences to make it possible to identify the cause in a specific patient. Look at the following charts to see the similarities; pay special attention to the differences of these important symptoms you could well see in your medical practice.

Bacterial Symptoms:

Symptoms	Staph Aureus	Campylo-bacter	E. Coli	Listeria	Salmonella	Botulism
Nausea	X			X		
Vomiting	X	X	X		X	
Abdominal Cramps	X	X	X		X	
Diarrhea	X	X	X	X	X	
Bloody Diarrhea		X	X			
Fever		X		X	X	
Dark Urine			X			
Stiff Neck				X		
Muscle Aches				X		
Joint Pain					X	
Constipation						X
Muscle Weakness						X

If the symptoms alone have not helped you isolate the specific bacteria infecting your patient, you might ask another sort of question, such as:
- Does anyone else in the family have similar symptoms?

- When did the family last eat at a restaurant?

- Have you prepared any unusual foods in your kitchen or used any unusual preparation methods?

You can see in the next chart that the incubation period (the time between contact with the organism and the appearance of symptoms) varies with the bacterial organism. The incubation period may vary from a few hours to a month, depending upon the organism.

Incubation Period

Bacterial Origin	Staph Aureus	Campylo-bacter	E.Coli	Listeria	Salmonella	Botulism
Incubation Period	1-6 hours	2-5 days	1-10 days	3-70 days	6-72 hours	3-30 days

Since your patient may have treated this illness as a case of the flu, and because most cases of food poisoning last only a few days, they may be starting to feel better by the time you see them in your office. On the other hand, they may feel sicker with each passing day. The duration of symptoms can help you identify the organism. The next chart compares the average duration of illness by bacteria type.

Duration of Illness

Bacterial Organism	Staph Aureus	Campylo-bacter	E.Coli	Listeria	Salmonella	Botulism
Duration of Illness	24-48 hours	2-10 days	5-10 days	1-7 days	5-7 days, or months	Several months

One of the best clues to help you determine the bacteria causing the infection could come from actually figuring out the food that created the problem. That information often comes from observing what the infected individuals ate that non-infected family members did not eat.

How does bacteria get into our food? Some bacteria live in the soil and actually grow on the fruits or vegetables we eat. Other bacteria live in the intestinal tracts of animals we consume. The **meat** we eat is the muscle of animals. Bacteria can contaminate the meat when the animal is processed at the slaughter house. Sometimes bird or animal feces can harbor the bacteria that contaminate meat and poultry. Bacteria can **inoculate** chicken eggs before the shell forms. Sea food can become contaminated with bacteria directly from ocean water. In some cases, foods are contaminated during preparation, especially in restaurants, if kitchen staff do not wash their hands adequately after using the toilet.

The following chart indicates the food types most associated with each food-borne bacteria.

Bacterial Sources of Food-borne Illness

Bacterial Source	Staph Aureus	Campylobacter	E. Coli	Listeria	Salmonella	Botulism
Milk/Dairy	X					
Raw Milk		X	X	X		
Eggs	X				X	
Meat	X		X		X	
Poultry	X	X			X	
Contaminated Water		X				
Raw fruits & Vegetables			X	X	X	
Deli meats & Hot dogs			X	X		
Sea food					X	
Toxin from Contaminated canned foods						X

At home appropriate safety precautions used when preparing food will reduce the chance of a food-borne infection. Do your best to ensure that your family and your patient's always wash their hands well before preparing foods in the kitchen. The U.S. Food and Drug Administration has a seven-step process on their website that home cooks can use to guard against food contamination.

Making the Diagnosis of bacterial foodborne illness

When all else fails, what test will provide the definitive identity of the cause of a foodborne illness? The pathogenic bacteria your patient ingested will continue through his or her entire gastrointestinal tract and end up in their **stools**. If you can obtain a sample of your patient's stool and send it to the laboratory, technicians can inspect it under a **microscope** and **culture** the bacteria for identification. Growing a culture may take a few days. This is often the method utilized to make the final diagnosis.

Botulism represents an exception to this process. If botulism is suspected a special test called the Mice Inoculation Test will make the diagnosis.

The **Mice Inoculation Test** proves very interesting, indeed. In the laboratory technicians inject the patient's blood or stool into two mice. They inject **antitoxin** to botulism toxin into one of the mice. If both mice survive, the patient does not have botulism. If the mouse not injected with antitoxin dies and the mouse injected with antitoxin survives, your patient has botulism. If both mice die, you should consider changing your business to a different lab. Patients with botulism can be sick for a long time and require intensive care to survive. These patients exhibit drooping eyelids and muscular weakness early on because the infection releases a toxin that paralyzes nerves and persists for weeks.

If your patient has started feeling better, it is still important to know the exact organism that made him or her sick. Yes! You must report incidents of food-

borne illness to the **Department of Health** so they can investigate and prevent others from becoming ill. We have experienced many large-scale foodborne illness outbreaks in our country, some from foods purchased at the market for home consumption, others at public eating establishments, especially fast-food restaurants. Such outbreaks around the world result in thousands of hospitalizations and hundreds of deaths each year. You can learn about major foodborne pathogen outbreaks that have occurred in the United States over the past several years by checking out this website:
http://www.cdc.gov/foodsafety/outbreaks/multistate-outbreaks/outbreaks-list.html

This next chart shows the recommended treatment of the foodborne illness once you have identified the responsible organism.

Treatment

Treatment	Staph Aureus	Campylobacter	E. Coli	Listeria	Salmonella	Botulism
Fluids	X	X	X	X	X	
Rest	X	X	X	X	X	
Antibiotics		X		X		
No Antibiotics	X		X		X	
Antitoxin						X

Food Preparation Guidelines

Patients need to understand how to prevent food-borne illness in their families. We mentioned previously the FDA seven-step recommendation for home cooks to avoid food-borne infections. The United States Department of Agriculture urges cooks to follow four basic rules:

1. Clean: Wash hands and surfaces often

2. Separate: keep meats and fruits/vegetables separated; don't cross contaminate

3. Cook: cook at the right temperature; don't eat undercooked food
4. Chill: refrigerate perishable foods immediately

The **Department of Agriculture** also provides a very detailed description of nine areas where you can protect yourself and family from foodborne pathogens. Look up the details at: http://www.fsis.usda.gov/foodsafety.

Those Pesky Viruses Also Want Some of the Action.

Foodborne illness can also have a viral origin. As you may recall, a virus is not considered a living organism; it doesn't contain all of the elements required for independent life. Instead, a virus attacks the DNA or RNA of its host organism (us) and causes our cells to replicate its virus structure until it burns out our cells such that no more virus cells are made. **Norovirus** causes more gastrointestinal illness that any other food-borne pathogen. Hepatitis A is another virus that can spread via the food-borne route.

When patients say they have "stomach flu," they commonly have Norovirus infection. Norovirus ranks as extremely contagious through exposure to **feces** or **vomit.** When someone in your house has stomach flu, everyone needs to wash their hands frequently to prevent the spread of that horrid illness. Norovirus can be spread from contaminated foods, door handles, eating utensils, and even clothing. Unfortunately, we have no vaccine and no definitive treatment for Norovirus. Even worse, patients can contract the illness over and over because Norovirus has multiple strains that can hide their identity from your immune system. Norovirus seems not to fight fairly at all.

Hepatitis A, another virus, can also spread via the food-borne route. Hepatitis A virus was a very contagious pathogen prior to the development of a vaccine. College parties provided a notorious venue for spreading Hepatitis A in years past. Fortunately, Hepatitis A infections are down about 90% as a result of the vaccine. Unlike Norovirus, Hepatitis A can only be contracted once, but it can

Medical Investigation 101

take up to six months for the disease to run its course. No one need experience Hepatitis A if they get vaccinated. College students would probably agree that getting a vaccination proves preferable to banning all college parties.

Below is a chart comparing Norovirus and Hepatitis A viruses.

Common Foodborne Viruses

Virus	Incubation Period	Duration of Illness	Source	Treatment	Vaccine	# Cases/ year U.S.
Norovirus	12 – 48 hours	1 – 3 days	Contact contamin-ation from vomit or stools	Fluids Rest Treat symptoms	None. Many strains	19 – 21 million per year
Hepatitis A	15 – 50 days	2 – 6 weeks	Food or water from infected person	Rest Treat symptoms	Yes	>250,000 per year

Norovirus and Hepatitis A have symptoms very similar to bacterial infections. Fortunately, Norovirus does not exhibit as many symptoms as Hepatitis A, as you can see in this chart.

Norovirus and Hepatitis A Symptoms

Symptoms	Norovirus	Hepatitis A
Diarrhea	X	X
Vomiting	X	X
Fatigue		X
Abdominal pain		X
Jaundice		X
Dark Urine		X

NOW, we must have covered EVERYTHING that can POSSIBLY cause a Food-borne Infection!

Not so fast there, Doc. Certain parasites can also cause illness when ingested in our water or foods. Parasites are one-celled, microscopic, living organisms that live in and damage their host. Cryptosporidium is the most common waterborne disease in the United States. **Toxoplasmosis** is the leading cause of foodborne death in the U.S. Other parasites that might cause your patients to request your help are Giardia, Cryposporidia, Cyclospora, and Trichinella. All are treatable, but most do not require treatment unless the host is **immune compromised**. As with bacterial foodborne illness, the diagnosis is generally made by microscopic stool examination. The symptoms and sources of parasite infections are shown in the following chart.

Water and Foodborne Parasites

Parasite	Cryptosporidia	Giardia	Cyclospora	Toxoplasma	Trichinella
Illness	Cryposporidlosis	Giardiosis	Cyclosporiasis	Toxoplasmosis	Trichinosis
Source	swimming pools, lakes	cats, dogs, deer, cattle, beavers	fecal contaminate food & water, imported produce	cat feces	under-cooked pork & wild game meat
Symptoms	watery diarrhea, cramps, nausea, vomiting, fever, weight loss	diarrhea, gas, greasy stools, nausea, vomiting, weight loss, dehydration	watery diarrhea, gas, fever, vomiting, weight loss, fatigue	mostly no symptoms unless pregnant; passed on to fetus	nausea, vomiting, diarrhea, fatigue, muscle pain

Have any of the foods you especially enjoy eating been involved in a large-scale food-borne illness? This next chart will answer that question, but you probably

Medical Investigation 101

will not need to change your favorite foods, unless you love drinking lake water. Lake water lovers probably need to expand their experience with other beverages.

Foods having recent history of pathogenic contamination outbreaks

Food type				
Fruits	Cantalopes	Cucumbers	Tomatoes	Pomegranate Seeds
Vegetables	Cilantro	Bean Sprouts	Lettuce	Spinach
Meats	Beef	Pork	Bologna	
Seafood	Shell fish	Tuna		
Poultry	Chicken			
Dairy	Raw Milk	Cheese	Ice Cream	
Nuts	Hazel Nuts	Pistachios	Peanuts	
Other	Cookie Dough	Caramel Apples	Lake Water	

After reading about all of the foods that can become contaminated with pathogens, you understand why so many of your patients will come to you for complaints about abdominal pain, fever, and diarrhea. Making the diagnosis requires asking questions, listening closely to your patients' stories, ordering appropriate tests, and determining what treatment will help alleviate the problem. Educating your patients about preventive measures they can take at home should prevent return visits for the same problem. The best physicians recognize that teaching can be just as important as treating!

Investigation 3.11B: Foodborne Pathogen Case

Grace is a 28-year-old female who presents in your office with complaints of recent onset abdominal cramps, diarrhea and vomiting, fever, and pain in her joints. Realizing the complaints are not specific to any particular illness, you are prepared to ask some questions and listen carefully to the responses.

Here is the conversation between you and Grace:

You: When did the symptoms begin?

Grace: I started having abdominal cramps early Wednesday morning. By noon I vomited and had a fever. That night I started having pain in my joints. It has been three days and I don't really feel any better. Do I have the flu?

You: The flu is a possibility. Has anyone else in the family had similar symptoms?

Grace: Well, yes. My boyfriend has similar symptoms that started at the same time. He is still sick as well, but he won't get up to come to see you.

You: That is interesting. I would not expect both you and your boyfriend to come down with the flu at exactly the same time. Usually one person begins to feel ill and then the next person feels sick a few days later. What types of foods did you eat in the days prior to feeling sick?

Grace: My boyfriend bought a rotisserie chicken at the market that didn't look quite as well cooked as I would have preferred. We ate it anyway; that was Monday evening. We ate a little later than planned, so the chicken sat out a few extra hours.

You: Well, Grace. This does sound like perhaps you and your boyfriend have a case of food poisoning. Your symptoms do not sound like you have a food-borne virus or parasite pathogen. Rather it sounds more like a bacterial origin. I am concerned that the chicken did not appear to be well cooked. Also, you said it sat out for several hours. This could well be the source of your illness. In order to know for sure, we need to send a specimen of your stool to the laboratory. They will conduct a microscopic examination and grow a culture to identify the exact organism. Then we will know whether prescribing an **antibiotic** will be helpful or not. In the meantime, I recommend you rest and drink lots of water so you don't become **dehydrated**.

This case represents a dangerous habit many people have adopted, leaving perishable foods out, unrefrigerated for extended periods of time. Consider developing these two good habits when you bring home a pre-cooked chicken:

1. Make sure the chicken is fully cooked; don't pick the lightest colored chicken in the batch. Also, look at the time stamp on the chicken; select one that has not been sitting out more than one hour.

2. When you get the chicken home, place it in the refrigerator immediately if you are not able to eat it right away.

Follow-up: As Grace's physician, you would call Grace to give her the results of the laboratory test. In this case you would also advise her that antibiotics are not recommended for this particular bacterial infection. You would then advise her that Salmonella illness usually lasts 5 to 7 days and ask her to contact you if she does not feel better in a few more days because Salmonella in some people can evolve into a more serious condition.

Investigation 3.12

3.12A: Head Injury
3.12B: The Eye

Investigation 3.12A: Head Injury

Introduction

You have now worked your way through quite a few medical cases using the process of information gathering, formation of a differential diagnosis, and then examining and testing to rule out possibilities until only the correct diagnosis remains. Does the practice of medicine always work that way? It does not. It does not in the same way that you will not make all the decisions you face in your life by considering all the possibilities and logically selecting the best one. Instead, our minds learn **patterns** and **routines** so that we can do complex tasks almost without thinking about them. A piano player first learns to read each note printed in a chord on the sheet of music, but after hours of practice his or her fingers seem to find each key automatically as the musician's eye scans rapidly across the shape of the printed chords.

The experienced healthcare professional similarly learns to see the patterns of many diseases and arrives at a diagnosis almost before finishing taking the history. That ability can enhance productivity, allowing the care provider to help more people. Alternatively, looking for a pattern can lead to mistakes when the mind jumps to a conclusion not completely supported by the facts. We must guard against our instincts, but also must pay attention to cues from our instincts that can sometimes guide us correctly when logic seems to fail. Getting the correct diagnosis every time takes a great deal of care and effort.

The Case

In today's case you are providing primary care, not in a hospital, not in an office, but in a gymnasium as part of your civic duty to support the local high school's sports program. You find yourself sitting on the bench of the Brent Hill High School's girls' varsity basketball team. The Cougars are currently undefeated. The bleachers are packed with wildly cheering parents and students, but you have an important job to do not associated with cheering for the home team. You have the responsibility of making sure any injuries during the basketball game receive prompt and proper attention. Playing sports helps young people grow strong bodies and minds, but competitive sports also create a risk of injury. You are saying to yourself, "Please let everyone stay healthy at today's game."

This particular game provides the home team spectators both excitement and frustration. Brent Hill's game plan starts out working well, but the rival team members have a game plan of their own. As the action moves into the final period, Brent Hill misses a few shots and finds itself suddenly six points behind. Alice Harper, a Brent Hill senior, has played hard all game, but as the final minutes tick away she feels a sense of desperation and knows she has to make something good happen. Playing defense, a careless pass by her opponent puts the basketball suddenly into her hands with no one between her and her team's basket. The fast break race begins. The rival team has two players close on Alice's heels as she races, dribbling the ball down the court.

As Alice leaps into the air to release her lay-up, four other outstretched hands reach up, hoping to tip that basketball away from its intended path into the hoop. The ball goes precisely where Alice hoped it would go, but simultaneously three young bodies blend into a single mass of arms and legs, dragged down ruthlessly by **gravity** and propelled forward out of control by **inertia**. As the team physician you miss completely the outcome of the shot because you are focused on those bodies flying through the air. Without even thinking, you find yourself running full speed down the polished basketball court with the full knowledge that the result of that much **kinetic energy** hitting the floor has to have unintended consequences.

You, plus two very experienced Brent Hill Paramedics whom you know well as Liz and Graham, arrive at the awkwardly entangled pile of girls splayed on the gymnasium floor. You cannot see much of Alice because the two girls who chased her down the court fell on top of her. You also do not see any **blood**, and you rejoice momentarily in that finding. Liz kneels at one side of the heap and Graham has gotten down on all fours at the other side to help untangle the players and begin to sort out any injuries. The two rival players are moving, cautiously, slowly, and groaning as they free themselves from the entanglement.

Paramedics receive extensive training in managing victims of trauma, so Liz and Graham have gone immediately into a practiced mode of trying to identify serious injuries quickly while not allowing the injured to do things that might make their situation worse. They caution the players not to move until they know more about their injuries.

At the same time your mind has focused on Alice because you know she hit the floor first with the combined inertia of three players, not one. She appeared at first to be shaking underneath the two other players. As Liz and Graham carefully help the top two players move away from Alice, you see that Alice's right leg has a distinct bend, not in a place normal legs bend. Alice is resting face down on the floor, no longer shaking, but not trying to get up. You look closer and are relieved to see respiratory movements. You bend down and call her name. No response.

Graham tells you that the two rival players appear to have no major injuries, and he suggests that he and Liz grab some supplies from their ambulance unit to stabilize that obviously broken leg prior to transporting Alice to the hospital.

As you learned previously, you are thinking circulation, airway, and breathing. What do you do to evaluate circulation and airway? (We noted respiratory movement already.)

You were happy to see that she fell with one arm elevated to protect her head from hitting the floor directly. There is no blood on her or the floor. No fractures of other bones are obvious. You see lots of good signs to suggest Alice did not receive any horrible injuries. What remains for you to consider in evaluating Alice?

If you are having trouble with that answer, why not take a history from Alice starting with her chief complaint. Oops. Alice is not responding to you!

Meanwhile Liz and Graham continue to apply their training and are recording Alice's vital signs. **Respiration** 28/minute. **Blood Pressure** 190/88. **Pulse** 140. You can see Alice's face and you lift her eyelids to examine her pupils. You see big **pupils** and almost no **iris** at all.

You turn to Liz and Graham and say, "Graham you support her legs, and I'll carry her upper body. Liz we are going to the hospital right now! Call ahead and tell them we have a closed head injury with a presumed **intracranial bleed** and need a **neurosurgeon** now."

Time for some physiology and an explanation: Of all the marvels of the human body, the human **brain** ranks right at the top. **Neurophysiologist**s, the scientists who study this organ, know a great deal about how it works but still have vast numbers of unanswered questions. You may be aware that trauma to the brain, especially from playing football, has received much debate in the media. Sports coaches increasingly sideline players who hit their heads for several weeks before allowing them to return to play. A blow to the head can bruise one or more areas of the brain with minimal symptoms, but without time to fully recover from that injury the brain has decreased **tolerance** to another injury.

The human body protects the brain by surrounding it with bone, the **skull**. In addition, the brain floats in a watery fluid called **cerebral spinal fluid** inside the skull as an extra protective cushion against **mechanical** injury. But the skull actually creates the potential for a type of injury you may not know about. Neurosurgeons (often referred to in slang as brain surgeons) will tell you that while they deal with many urgent problems in their practice, they only have one condition they deem a true emergency (a problem they need to treat without any delay). An **intracranial arterial bleed** constitutes that single emergency in neurosurgery. If an artery is bleeding inside the skull, the skull bone confines that blood so that the pressure inside the skull climbs to the pressure in the artery. Normally the **veins** inside the skull would drain away the blood so the pressure would not rise, but when an artery has broken open that no longer happens as the blood leaves its normal path from arteries flowing into veins.

If the pressure inside the skull grows to match the arterial blood pressure, the flow of blood and oxygen to the brain comes to a halt and brain cells cannot survive very long in that condition. In this case presentation we have distracted you, Liz, and Graham with an obviously broken leg, but we wanted you to recognize that Alice was not moving or talking, so the real emergency did not come from a broken leg, but from an injury to the head. We had you look at the pupils that were abnormally dilated, and that finding signaled that the brain no longer was sending signals to the eyes. We put words in your mouth to declare Alice's condition a life-threatening emergency that required immediate action in a hospital from a neurosurgeon.

The idea of performing surgery on either the heart or the brain appears to have come to medicine relatively recently. History calls Dr. Harvey **Cushing** the Father of Modern Neurosurgery for his creation of methods to treat the brain surgically beginning about the time of the First World War (early 1900s). Having said that, a procedure called **trephination** dates back to around 6500 BCE and appears to represent one of the earliest forms of surgery. Trephination means cutting a hole into the skull, not actually surgery on the brain but an important procedure for our injured basketball-player. Alice needs an emergency life-saving trephination to relieve the high pressure inside her skull so that normal blood flow to her brain can resume. A modern neurosurgeon does this very carefully with specially designed tools in order to relieve that pressure safely under **sterile** conditions (to avoid any infection). In addition, a modern

neurosurgeon would next find the site of bleeding (surgery on the brain itself) and treat that as well.

Why might Alice's fall have caused a bleed inside her head while the other players did not have similar serious injury? Alice might have hit her head on the floor with enough force to actually **fracture** her skull to produce that injury, but our view of the event actually suggested that did not happen. She actually appeared to protect her head with her hand as she fell. This may have been consistent with a **concussion**, but her injury symptoms went beyond a concussion. Alice suffered a more severe injury because she had a **cerebral aneurysm**, a weak or thin area in the wall a blood vessel in the brain that occurs in about 1 in every 10,000 people. As a result, she was more likely than others to have that vessel break open inside her skull without warning.

Rapid diagnosis of this event, along with the prompt action you, Liz, and Graham took to get Alice to a neurosurgeon quickly, saved her life.

Case Review:

This case represents a departure from our normal process of collecting information and moving methodically to a diagnosis and then treatment. Instead we have a case of an emergency in which medical training made it possible to make quick evaluations and move right to life-saving treatment. Some fields of medicine commonly put providers in emergency situations, while others rarely involve the need to make quick decisions and take prompt action.

Make a list of the following specialties on a piece of paper. After each one, write RARELY or COMMONLY to indicate the frequency you would expect that specialty to encounter an emergency that requires decisive treatment in the next few minutes.

Medical Investigation 101

Medical Specialty

1. CARDIOLOGIST
2. DERMATOLOGIST
3. EMERGENCYROOM PHYSICIAN
4. OBSTETRICIAN
5. PATHOLOGIST
6. PODIATRIST
7. ANESTHESIOLOGIST
8. ORTHOPEDIST
9. OPTHAMOLOGIST
10. TRAUMA SURGEON

Take a moment to think about your own personality and ask yourself if you think you would find a career that presented you with desperate emergencies energizing or exhausting. Careers that deal with emergencies exist in many forms not always associated with medicine, for example policemen and firemen. People who elect to fill those careers provide services of great value to society as a whole. Your perspective on this issue can easily change as you grow and have new experiences. Do not make any lasting decisions; just consider your current feelings, briefly, today.

Alice experienced a severe injury because she had a condition that made that injury more likely. She did not cause that condition or even know she had an **aneurysm**. That hardly seems fair, and yet such things exist in the world. In many ways medical science represents a desire to restore some fairness to nature, by allowing people who have injury or disease, through no fault of their own, to have their health restored. The desire to make the world fairer for every person can serve as a reason to elect a career in healthcare.

Take a moment to think about anything you want to remember about your feelings regarding Alice's injury and the role of those who worked hard to restore her to a normal life.

We might note that Alice had just run at top speed down the basketball court, so we would expect her pulse rate to register high compare to her resting pulse rate. We would expect a rapid respiration rate from that exercise also. What about blood pressure? The high pulse rate might make her blood pressure rise, but the arteries feeding blood to her muscles would be dilated wide open to get lots of blood flow and oxygen to the muscles that were working so hard. So we might expect a mild rise in blood pressure.

Normal Vital Signs Review:

We found unusual vital signs for Alice immediately after her fall. She had an elevated pulse rate and a quite high blood pressure. Before we look again at Alice's values, we can review normal values for each of these.

Blood Pressure

Systolic Blood Pressure: Normal resting systolic pressure in a young adult is below 120 mmHg.

Diastolic Blood Pressure: Normal resting diastolic pressure in a young adult is below 80 mmHg

Strenuous activity can increase both systolic and diastolic blood pressure.

Heart Rate

Normal resting heart rate is between 60 and 100 beats per minutes. Trained athletes are usually at the lower end of the spectrum.

Respirations

Normal resting respiratory rate is between 12 and 20 breaths per minute.

Strenuous activity can raise the respiratory rate.

Liz and Graham found for Alice, 28 breaths per minute, a blood pressure of 190/88 millimeters of mercury, and a pulse rate of 140 beats per minute. Those vital signs represent something much more than strenuous exercise. Alice had those signs because her brainstem was telling her heart and her arteries that her brain was not getting enough blood supply to stay alive. Those vital signs amplified the message that Alice needed a very fast trip to the hospital to see a neurosurgeon. And the neurosurgeon needed to lower the pressure inside Alice's skull very quickly to save her life.

Medical Investigation 101

In case you are interested in our rating of medical specialties based on their frequency of emergency encounters, you can find our score card below:

| 1 – C | 3 – C | 5 – R | 7 – C | 9 – R |
| 2 – R | 4 – C | 6 – R | 8 – R | 10-C |

Investigation 3.12B: The Eye

In the preceding case, the marker of the problem of greatest concern lay in finding the pupils fixed and dilated. But what exactly is the "pupil," and what makes it normally dilate and constrict in response to the level of light in the room?

In the following diagram of the eye, we have numbered the major parts and then connected those numbers to the name of that structure. Compare the numbers in the diagram with the key below to identify the main parts of the eye.

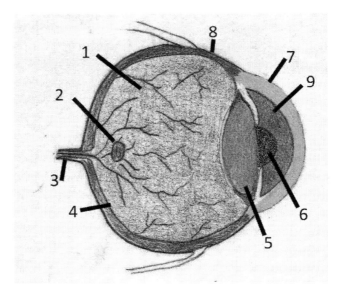

Suppose Alice is visiting an art museum and looking at a painting of a magnifying glass. A ray of light from the museum lighting reflects from the lovely oil painting, and bounces towards Alice's eyes. Magically that ray of light ends up allowing Alice's mind to enjoy the beauty of that oil painting. Let's talk about how that miracle comes about, going step by step.

Cornea

Light reflected from the piece of art travels all about the room, but the light Alice sees first contacts Alice at her **cornea**. The cornea is a **transparent** layer of tissue that covers the front of the eye. It protects the iris and lens from the outside world, keeping out dust and microbes in the air while also keeping the fluids in the eye from leaking out. The cornea plays a role in gathering or turning light in toward the lens of the eye directly under the cornea. The cornea has a fixed geometry, while the lens can change its shape to bring images to a sharp focus inside the eye.

<u>Eye Diagram Key</u>
1 = Fovea
2 = Macula
3 = Optic Nerve
4 = Retina
5 = Lens
6 = Pupil
7 = Cornea
8 = Sclera
9 = Iris

A very uniform symmetric shape of the cornea is important to its ability to allow light onto the lens without introducing any distortion. A misshaped cornea will prevent the lens from creating a clear image. Modern medicine has devised methods of reshaping the cornea to remove such defects commonly classified as **astigmatism**. Beginning in the 1980's **radial keratotomy** (RK) surgery was introduced to make these corrections. In this procedure a tiny scalpel or knife controlled by a surgeon peering through a binocular microscope makes small cuts into the cornea to correct myopia, or nearsightedness caused by an abnormally shaped cornea. Since 2002 **Lasik** surgery has provided eye surgeons a better tool to improve patients' vision. In Lasik surgery a laser makes the cuts precisely to allow reshaping of the cornea to correct **myopia** (near-sightedness), **hyperopia** (far-sightedness), and **astigmatism**. (You will visualize the eye deformity causing myopia and hyperopia a little later.)

Medical Investigation 101

Your eye lid slams shut very rapidly to protect the delicate surface of the cornea from impending trauma. If something does strike the cornea, damage occurs quite easily. We call a minor injury to the surface of the cornea a **corneal abrasion**. Such an abrasion can easily occur should dust, sand, wood or metal get into your eye, and cause small scratches on the surface of the cornea. Superficial scratches usually heal in a day, but deep scratches can scar and potentially permanently affect vision. Persistently painful injuries to an eye deserve a trip to an urgent care facility for evaluation and treatment. Don't risk permanent injury.

Iris

After passing through the cornea, light reaches the **iris**. The iris is that pigmented, or colored, part of your eye so important in romantic poetry. The black looking hole in the iris we call the pupil. The iris stops or absorbs light. The pupils allow the light to pass into the inner eye globe.

A few words about the color of our eyes. In some eyes the iris appears blue, in others green or brown. Babies virtually always start life with blue eyes. By the time the baby becomes a teenager, blue eyes have become the least common eye color. For a baby's eyes to remain blue into adulthood, the baby must have only blue-eye genes, two of them, because that gene we classify as recessive. Green and brown eye color comes from genes we classify as dominant, meaning we need only one of them to dictate the eye color. Rarely, you might see a person with irises that appear pink. In that case the color comes from their blood vessels, because they lack any pigment in their irises.

When someone compliments your beautiful brown eyes, they are actually complimenting the color of your iris and not really the color of your eye. When the poet says your eyes act as windows into your soul, he or she is no longer talking about anatomy or physiology. The location of the human soul goes far beyond the scope of *Medical Investigation 101*. We expect that topic might be covered in *Medical Investigation 947*.

Your iris is shaped like a donut, like a glazed donut, not a jelly filled one. The iris opens and closes to control the amount of light passing through. In bright light conditions the iris gets smaller, or contracts, to allow less light into your eye. In dim light conditions the iris opens, or dilates, to allow in more light. Commands to dilate or contract come from inside the brain. If you shine a bright light into only one eye, both pupils will become very small, so the decision comes from a part of the brain that has begun to integrate information coming from both eyes. Alice's eyes dilated because her brain cells involved in controlling her pupils were no longer functioning properly.

The Pupil

Light from the world about us passes through the cornea, and if too bright gets cut down by the iris allowing the right amount to enter through the pupil. What is the pupil? It's simply the open space in the center of the iris through which light passes headed for the retina at the back of the eye. The pupil doesn't dilate or contract, even though people often say "her pupil is contracted or dilated". Instead of saying "the pupil is dilated", to be accurate we should be saying "the iris is dilated". The pupil is just a void or hole in the center of the iris.

Lens

Light passing through the pupil enters the **lens**. If you recall, the cornea bends light toward the lens. The lens further bends the light such that all the light reflected from a single point on the art work that reaches the lens meets at a single point in focus on the retina. In the study of physics, you will learn that the light changes its direction of travel inside the lens because the lens material actually decreases the velocity of the light slightly. Reflected light from objects in front of us is spreading out as it comes to us, but the lens turns that light back together so that the light energy from a single spot out in our field of view comes back together at a single spot on the surface of the retina in our eye. The lens changes its shape to focus the light from a specific distance depending on the object we choose to see most clearly. As we age, beginning for most people around age 40, our lens begins losing its flexibility, and thus its ability to focus equally on nearby and faraway objects. It may become necessary to have reading glasses for near vision or **bifocals**, which have two corrections, one for reading and the other for distance vision. Unfortunately, the eyes of a large number of people throughout the world have less than perfect vision; in fact, it is estimated that nearly 40% of the world population is myopic (near-sighted). Professional baseball players must have exceptional vision in order to hit a 95 mile-per-hour cut fast-ball. For those of us in the more normal category of vision we may have to pin our hopes on different careers.

Cataract describes a **progressive** condition in which the lens in the eye grows cloudy, starting in the center and expanding outward over time. Sun glasses that reduce ultraviolet rays may slow this progression, but it appears that cataracts eventually develop. Cataracts constitute the most common cause of loss of vision around the world in those over the age of 40. By age 80 half of all Americans have cataracts or they have had a very sophisticated, quick surgical procedure to remove the cataract and replace it with an artificial lens.

Retina

The **retina** functions as the movie screen of the eye. It sits at the back of the eye and forms the surface upon which the lens focuses the light images that give us vision. **Myopia** describes a condition where the lens focuses the light beam in front of the retina. **Hyperopia** describes the opposite condition, where the beam is not yet focused when the light hits the retina and would need to have more distance to come into focus. In the images below the smaller magnifying glass represents the point of focus in myopia (left), normal vision (center) and hyperopia (far-sightedness, right).

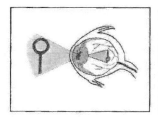 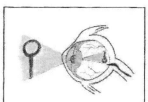 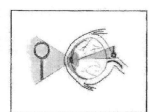

There are three important things to notice in the diagrams above:

1. The base of the smaller cone represents the point of focus in each condition.
2. Eye shape differs slightly in each condition, altering the relationship between lens and retina
3. Images are displayed on the retina inverted from their actual orientation in life. Our brain turns the image upright without our awareness.

The retina is a complex and fragile structure of ten layers having light sensitive cells including rods and cones. **Rods** are photoreceptor cells concentrated at the **peripheral** edges of the retina and used for peripheral vision in less intense light. **Cones** are responsible for our color vision and work best in relatively bright light conditions. It is estimated that each eye has about 7 million cone receptors in three colors: around 64% are red receptors, 32% green receptors, and about 2% are blue receptors. These three receptor types work together so you can see all of the blended variations of our kaleidoscopic world of color.

In order to perceive a nice, clear picture your lens must focus the image onto a smooth layer of receptors. Things can go wrong within the retina. The retina can detach from the posterior surface of the eye; a **detached retina** is an urgent medical condition that must be treated within a couple of days or permanent loss of vision can result in that eye.

The retina is well supplied with small blood vessels. The condition of those vessels can indicate overall vascular health and because the retina is transparent, physicians can inspect these vessels more than any others. To do this they use a small hand-held instrument called an **ophthalmoscope**. Diabetes causes changes in the blood vessels that can be seen readily during an eye examination with that device. Small vessel disease of the retina from diabetes can disrupt vision, a common complication of diabetes.

Medical Investigation 101

When we look directly at a specific object, for example a word we are reading, our eyes place the image of that word in a special small region of the retina, a region densely packed with cones, making our vision of that word extremely acute. That region we call the macula. Older individuals can suffer progressive failure of the macula called **macular degeneration.** We have no cure for macular degeneration but ophthalmologists can now provide treatment that slows the progression of this condition.

Optic Nerve (and Where it Goes)

Traditionally health care providers have called the connection of the retina to the brain Cranial Nerve II. Today we know that Cranial Nerve II, usually called the Optic Nerve, is not really a nerve at all. It differs in structure from the other nerves in our body. We should think of this nerve as being a part of our brain reaching into the back of each eye. Brain neurons in this structure come together inside the skull in a "node" called the Optic Chiasm, and then divide again to form two channels or tracks going back to the region of our brain at the back of our head. The majority of brain cells in the cortex of our brain participate in vision. Understanding and interpreting what we are seeing probably represents the most amazing task our brain can perform. Some would even say all of our creativity is visual. Even composers say that they see the music they create. Our dreams and imagination appear to have vision as their basis. Our eyes allow us to accurately recognize hundreds of faces of our family and friends. Probably not by accident do we communicate our understanding of a complex issue by saying, "I see what you mean."

Glaucoma

The eyeball or globe is filled with a clear watery fluid called **aqueous humor.** Cells in one part of the eye constantly make this fluid and it is absorbed back into the blood stream in a different area close to the edge of the iris. If something disrupts this absorption, the pressure inside the eye can become elevated and cause damage to the neurons in the retina that carry our visual information into our brain. Eye doctors can measure this pressure and have several methods to treat this condition we call **glaucoma.**

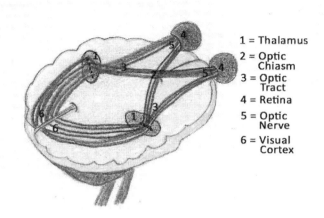

1 = Thalamus
2 = Optic Chiasm
3 = Optic Tract
4 = Retina
5 = Optic Nerve
6 = Visual Cortex

Occipital Lobe

After a quick stop at the **thalamus**, our visual signals journey into the **occipital lobes**. You now understand that we do not really see with our eyes. Our eyes collect information about the light reflected from objects around us and that information we ship to the occipital lobes. Neural networks in the occipital lobes allow us to understand and recognize what we see. Your occipital lobes work in conjunction with your temporal lobes to store images and thus create your visual memories. Without a temporal lobe, everyday would be a new day at school or anywhere else you go. Every TV show, every video game would be full of new images because you wouldn't remember having ever seen them before. You would walk right by your best friends because you wouldn't remember what they look like.

The loss of vision, blindness, represents a huge disability we have difficulty understanding if our eyes work normally. Individuals who must deal with blindness often prove truly amazing in what their minds can accomplish. We do not fully understand how our brains go about repurposing themselves, but it would appear that in many cases the occipital lobe takes on different roles in the minds of individuals who cannot see. Even the blind have been heard to say, "Yes, I see."

Eye Activity 1: Simulate Blindness for 10 minutes with a Partner

Directions:

1. Blindfold yourself or have your partner blindfold you.
2. Make sure you cannot see anything; come on, don't cheat.
3. See if you can make it 10 minutes without your vision. Move carefully around as you try to maneuver around the room. Use your other senses to compensate for your lack of sight and stay safe.
4. Your partner's job is to make sure you don't get hurt.
5. After 10 minutes, remove the blindfold.
6. Now it's your partner's turn.
7. Repeat steps 1 through 5

Investigation 3.13

3.13A: The Brain
3.13B: Normal or Abnormal?

Investigation 3.13A: The Brain

In the previous chapter your patient's pupils were dilated and did not respond to light as she lay on the basketball court. You learned that this finding did not represent an injury to her eyes. Instead, it indicated that the patient's brain was not responding normally to the stimulation of a bright light shone into her eyes. A person's eyes and brain must work together to provide them the ability to see the wonderful world around them because vision requires much more than simply the detection of light. The brain must process the patterns of light that fall on the retina to create a mental model and an understanding of what that image represents. That task constitutes an amazingly complex achievement.

Anatomists study the structure of the human, starting with the large structures we can easily see, and going down to the structures so tiny that we can only examine them with the aid of an electron microscope. Anatomists who specialize in studying the brain we call **Neuroanatomists.**

You probably know very well the meaning of the word "**gross**." Actually, that word has several different meanings: the one you do not want applied to anything you do or say, one that often refers to the total salary one gets paid before any deductions, and in medical science a third meaning that indicates a structure big enough to be seen and studied simply by looking at it. Below you will find a drawing of the gross anatomy of the brain.

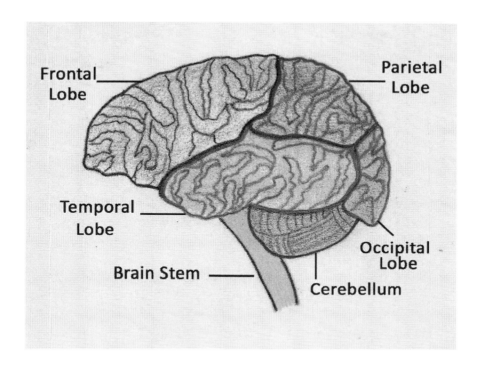

This view of the brain looks inside the skull of a head from the left side (**profile**) with the nose pointing off to your left. Later you will see another view of the brain looking down on it, as if you were on a ladder looking down from on high at a person standing directly below you. From that position you can see that the human brain is divided down the middle into left and right halves. The neuroanatomist would call each half a **hemisphere** (hemi- meaning half and – sphere meaning a ball). We each have a left hemisphere and a right hemisphere of our brain inside our head.

The neuroanatomist further divides the human brain into four sections, called **lobes**, in each hemisphere. These four lobes all have a similar surface appearance, almost looking like they are composed of a ball of heavy smooth rope all tangled up. That tangled rope surface they call the **cerebral cortex,** and they divide it into the **frontal, parietal, temporal, and occipital lobes.** An additional region of the brain has different surface appearance as if made up of a ball of much smaller rope, the **cerebellum.**

If you study the anatomy of an organ like the heart, you can look at its structure and almost immediately understand what it does and how it functions to pump blood. The brain does not cooperate at all with that approach to understanding how it works because this organ does not perform a **mechanical** function. The cells that do the work inside the brain use **electro-chemical** processes, not mechanical. So we get very little understanding of how the brain works by studying its outward appearance, which we have now learned to call the brain's **gross anatomy**. Nonetheless, these diagrams of the brain have given you a basic view of the brain's anatomy.

We can dig a little deeper into this topic by trying to categorize the role each lobe seems to play in the many jobs our brain performs. As we do that, you probably should not totally believe the descriptions you will read. The more we know about the brain, the more we believe that no two brains think completely alike.

We know clearly that very young children who suffer some form of head injury that destroys a particular area of the brain, surprisingly appear to grow older with amazingly normal brain function. Physicians common describe this ability of the brain by the term "**neural plasticity**," suggesting that the brain's **neurons** have the ability to "learn" and "adapt" to meet the individual's needs regardless of where they sit inside the brain. In other words, when we say a particular section of the brain does a specific task, we may find normal individuals with a different location for that brain activity.

The traditional way of teaching students about the brain consisted of assigning names to all the various regions of turns and twists in the brain's surface. Next, the student learned names for all the structures inside the brain seen by looking at photographs of stained, cross-sectional slices through the brain. Students could easily find themselves memorizing bizarre sounding words that name dozens upon dozens of shapes and features of the brain's gross anatomy.

Finally, students memorized the apparent roles these structures play in the workings of the brain, as identified by the observations of scientists over centuries of the deficits exhibited by people who have injuries to those parts of their brain.

More recently, sophisticated scanners using **radioisotopes** have allowed scientists to observe increased activity in various parts of the brain in living research subjects as they think about various topics or questions, so that researchers can increase our knowledge of where various mental activities appear to take place inside this organ. This quest has value in allowing **neurologists** or **neurosurgeons** to know where to look for brain damage when faced with a patient with a specific constellation of symptoms, but this approach probably will not give you any important insight how your brain does all the amazing things it can do. So, in this book we are not going to burden you with basal ganglia, the medulla oblongata, the cingulate gyrus, or the telodiencephalic sulcus. I hope you will forgive us.

Before we move on, we do want you to have an awareness that a very common cause of death and permanent disability, especially in older individuals, comes from a blockage of an artery in the brain or a rupture of a blood vessel in the brain that causes a region of the brain to stop working. We call such an event a **stroke**. Fortunately, if we recognize a stroke and get the victim to a stoke-center hospital quickly, the effects of the stroke can often be reversed. If you are with someone who has a rapid loss of speech, or loss of sensation or movement on one side of their body, think immediately that they may have had a stroke and do your best to get them transported to a hospital immediately. Getting treatment quickly makes a huge difference in the **outcome** of such an event. Everyone should have the ability to recognize the symptoms of a stroke so they can respond correctly to such an emergency. Your recognition of these symptoms and prompt response could save the life of someone you love.

Medical Investigation 101

Put on Your Seat Belt for a Whirlwind Tour of the Lobes of the Brain

We are not going deeply into brain anatomy, but we want you to have the basics.

As its name suggests, the **frontal lobe** sits right behind your forehead. We often say one's personality emanates from the frontal lobe. Your emotions, your determination, your passions, your hopes appear to live in this lobe. Neurosurgeons, who treat patients who have injured their frontal lobes in an automobile accident, notice that such individuals often appear to recover fully by all standard objective nervous system examination criteria, and yet they no longer seem to interact with others as they did before their injury or achieve the goals in life everyone expected of them. We, therefore, see the frontal lobe as playing a **modulating** role in the subtle, unique skills and traits that make us who we are.

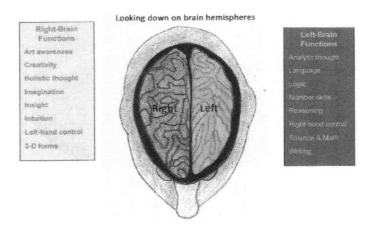

The **parietal lobes** are located on the upper sides of your head above your ears in both hemispheres. The parietal lobes seem to have an invisible, distorted diagram of your entire body drawn on its surface, such that stimulation of any point in that part of the brain evokes a sensation of something touching that part of your body. These distorted diagrams constructed by neuroanatomists we call a **cortical homunculus**. Actually, we have two of these neurologic maps across each parietal lobe, one associated with **sensation** and one **motor** (muscle movement).

So, think of the parietal lobe of the brain as the highest level of sensory and motor awareness of all your body's sensations and movement. The left side of the body maps to the right side of the brain, and the right side of the body maps to the left hemisphere of the brain. This apparent cross wiring of the brain occurs consistently throughout the animal kingdom, and scientists have put forward a variety of theories for this crossed-up wiring. You can think up your own theory if you like.

The **temporal lobe** manages your hearing and speech. The temporal lobe seems to allow you to understand and comprehend what you hear. The temporal lobe also appears to play a role in putting a name to objects that we see.

The **occipital lobe** is located at the back of your head and it processes the visual input coming from our eyes. Recall we mentioned that the optic nerve was incorrectly named and should be considered part of the brain. The retina actually begins processing visual images and actually throws away over 90% of the information continuously registered by the rods and cones. Layers and layers of neurons in the occipital lobe of the brain continue the process of recognizing visual features that finally allow us to recognize that a piano looks different from a dog.

The **cerebellum** does not officially count as a lobe of your brain, but it has a very important function sitting down low, back there behind your ears. The cerebel um manages the **coordination** of all the muscle movements of your body. When you go to catch a ball, the cerebellum figures out exactly what a dozen muscles need to do, and when, to get that job done. If you decide to write your name, the cerebellum apparently figures out every tiny little movement of your fingers needed to make that happen. Awesome does not begin to cover the talents of the cerebellum.

One more part of the brain deserves mentioning. The **brain stem,** tucked below the cerebellum at the top of the spinal cord, seems to have command of all those things your body needs to do that you do not have time to think about. It remembers, without being asked, to keep you breathing, to crank up the right activities in your stomach and intestines to digest your lunch, to get your heart cranked up for the big game, and probably to suggest to your brain that you take off that heavy coat on a hot day.

Now for the Really Important Stuff

What's really going on between your ears? Medical science has struggled with that question for centuries and most would agree we still know very little. Having said that, one can safely bet the coming decades will vastly improve our understanding of how the brain really works. The quest for that understanding has taken scientists in a very different direction than you might expect.

Recall that the brain does its work electrochemically inside cells. The cells in the brain communicate with each other by way of action potentials. The cells can generate a pulse of electrical current, known as an **action potential**, that travels down the long "arms" or "legs" that branch out from the cell and eventually touch the surface of other brain cells. We usually think of the cells in our body as being very, very tiny, yet nerve cells have these tiny "arms" that can extend a considerable distance, even many inches. Did I mention that we have many billions of these cells inside our brain? We do. And we have different types of brain cells, and we have some cells in our nervous system that appear to act as **insulators**, just as we use insulators in electrical circuits to make sure signals only go where we want them to go.

Not long after the discovery of the microscope, anatomists recognized that cells in the brain appeared to form layers with a tangle of "arms" (**axons** and **dendrites**) going in all directions between layers. A neuroscientist named Warren McCulloch wrote a paper in 1943 with a mathematician, Water Pitts, first suggesting how neurons work together to form **neural networks**. **Alan Turing**, an important early pioneer in digital computing at the time, became fascinated by these early drawings showing the cellular organization of the brain and recognized that neural networks were indeed "self-organizing" computers.

He too began to imagine the ways these interactions created logic and allowed humans to learn.

Today computer scientists working with models of neural networks are generating new insight into our understanding of the way our central nervous system has evolved to allow us to shape and understand our environment. It appears that our genetics **differentiates** cells that multiply and interconnect during **fetal** development, but these interconnections grow and adapt throughout our lives. Each neuron in the network decides when to create an action potential in response to the action potentials that other neurons send through their "arms" to its surface. Each brain neuron, over time, can modify the contribution from each input "arm" even to make some inputs have a negative effect they call **inhibition**. The **weighted** combination of action potentials reaching a neuron in the brain determine when that neuron generates its own action potential that it sends to other neurons. The ability of neurons to gradually change the importance of the various inputs it receives allows the neural network to improve its performance or "**learn**."

The manner in which the neurons decide how to adjust their sensitivity to inputs scientists call **backpropogation.** Backpropogation has become a sophisticated topic in mathematics and clearly a key to our understanding of how our brain works. In addition, backpropogation also has importance in the quest in computer science to create **artificial intelligence** and smart robots. The appreciation of the way the cells in our brain communicate and adjust their communication constitutes the real essence for each of us to begin to understand this incredible organ, much more important than our learning the names of all the anatomical features of the brain.

Brittany Wenger, as a teenager in 2013, created a computer program capable of diagnosing breast cancer from **aspiration biopsy** data better than traditional methods of examination of this data. Brittany used a "neural network" program that taught itself how to detect cancer based on training itself using thousands of examples taken from hospital data libraries. How does this work? Hospital data has specific sets of observations that we might label a, b, c, d…. x, y, z. For each one of these sets of findings for a particular patient we know that they eventually were found either to have a cancer or not. Suppose we think of observations "a through z" as action potentials for individual brain neurons that land on a single neuron we will call neuron Bill in the brain. We want to make Bill into the world's best evaluator of breast cancer. To do that Bill needs to know when a specific set of "a through z" inputs actually indicates cancer. So we are going to guess that Bill should signal cancer if the sum of weighted inputs "a through z" totals more than 100. We need then to find a unique weighting for each input that will make Bill an expert, if it indeed exists.

Brittany started out with a guess for all the weights, but as her computer looked at each case from the hospital data libraries the neural network program adjusted each weight using a backpropogation scheme. The backpropogation scheme essentially looked at each new data sample and asked if a tiny increment in every weight would make Bill's decision better or worse at knowing the right answer. It would then add a tiny step to the apparently best weighting factor to improve Bill's performance. You can think of this as the way you might go about finding the top of a hill you are standing on if blindfolded. You could move your foot around in all directions until you find a direction that appears to move you upward the most and take a step in that direction. Then you would test again and take another step.

Brittany's first effort failed to achieve a solution that worked on new sets of data. She had to **reconfigure** the way she organized the data and start over. Finally, she found a weighting that did give the right answer with an amazingly high accuracy.

The human brain has billions of neurons attached to each other in neural networks that are constantly adjusting themselves in a similar manner. The basic construct of the network appears to arise in our **genetic blueprint**, but the weighting of the interconnections, indeed the **density** of the interconnections appears to result from the experience and activities of each brain. When one person spends thousands of hours moving their fingers up and down the neck of a banjo playing bluegrass tunes, they refine neural networks very different from the person who spends a similar amount of time swinging a baseball bat at a curve ball, or practicing a foreign language, or animating a funny cartoon.

That's what scientists are learning about our brain, and as we learn more, we are going to get better at teaching, and we are going to get better at figuring out how to help our brains work more efficiently and make fewer errors. Google has reported that it has pretty much finished its mission of retrieving information for people, and next it wants to start helping people think in new and powerful ways. Now that's exciting!

You have probably heard the old adage, "To err is human." Humans cannot seem to avoid making mistakes. When we explained backpropogation as having a similarity to finding the top of a hill by testing each step, we also illustrated a limitation of neural networks because that backpropogation scheme would take you to the top of the hill you start out on, but not get you to the top of the nearby mountain, because to get there you would need first to go downhill and then back up. The neural networks in our brain have shortcomings we commonly label as fatigue, distraction, overloading, and forgetting. We cannot overcome these with diligence or training or eating the right diet. But as we increasingly understand the limitation of our mind, we have the power to develop methods that bridge the gaps to our shortcomings. That is happening all around us even today. Jet fighter pilots do not have fast enough reflexes to fly their planes, so engineers have developed controls that make it possible for the pilot to decide where to go and leave the details to the plane. Similar systems will eventually take over automobile driving and many other tasks in our lives that make us safer and more successful.

Investigation 3.13B: Normal or Abnormal?

We have previously noted that the educational pathway to becoming a physician stretches over many years. But one navigates that journey only one day at a time. Even after one completes medical school and specialty training (called a residency), physicians continue to study to remain up-to-date with the latest information and innovations in their field. That never-ending quest for knowledge would seem too heavy a burden except that the rewards of a career restoring good health to others make the effort worthwhile.

The Case Setting

On this Friday evening your role, experiencing different aspects of a career in medical science, sends you to the airport to fly off to a medical conference for the weekend, a symposium that will teach you new concepts to apply in your practice. You have arranged for another physician to cover any emergencies your patients might encounter while you attend the conference.

This trip might feel like a holiday except that this morning you awoke to a freezing cold house. Something you may have learned about life is that a broken furnace never happens when you have time to deal with it; things like plumbing appear to always decide to break down when you have no spare time to deal with them. Fortunately, you were able to reach your heating system repairman when you got to the office this morning, and he called you back in the early afternoon to say he fixed the problem by replacing a bad thermostat. Your old thermostat was not calling for heat from the furnace when the temperature in the house fell below normal.

As you now settle into your airplane seat before takeoff, your mind dwells on that thermostat. That thermostat could have ruined your trip. Whoever thinks about thermostats? They just sit there patiently on the wall keeping our homes warm in winter and cool in the summer. Thermostats keep the house temperature "normal."

As you see patients in your medical practice you constantly check all manner of things related to their body and health to see if they appear normal or abnormal. When a physician finds something abnormal that finding becomes a clue in the search for a diagnosis that we hope leads to a treatment. Noting elements of the history and physical examination that appear normal also contribute to reaching the correct diagnosis. We have come to understand that path to a diagnosis in medicine very clearly, but that broken thermostat serves as a reminder of a very important principle that lies behind that methodology. We might define that principle by saying, "Normal does not happen by accident!" Anything we measure, or test, or examine in medicine, anything that we evaluate as normal or abnormal, has some physiologic mechanism that controls that feature. "Normal does not happen accidently!"

[If your love of science happens, especially, to favor physics, you might view these comments about "normal" findings as having a parallel to the difficult to understand concept of entropy in thermodynamics. Physicists would say that one must do work to create and maintain order. Biological systems appear to also obey the spirit of that edict and must do work to keep things "normal."

The furnace does not come on to heat a house accidently. The **thermostat** must sense that the temperature in the house has fallen before a set value and must then signal the furnace to send heat. That series of steps keeps the house at its normal temperature. When the house temperature became abnormal the repairman found the problem did not come from a broken furnace, but from a broken thermostat.

Engineers who design controllers define a **closed loop system** as one that measures its output, compares that measurement to a set point (the desired output), and then uses the difference between the two to dictate what happens next. An **open loop system** would have set inputs but no measure of the output, so the system would have no ability to compensate for any external factors. If you had an open loop heating system in your house, you would expect the house to get too warm on a warm day and feel cold on a cold day.

When you get the flu and your body temperature goes much higher than its normal value of close to 98.6 degrees Fahrenheit, would you say that your furnace has gone wild or has your thermostat failed? Circle your guess about the bad element:

FURNACE or THERMOSTAT

Do you actually have a furnace and a thermostat inside your body? You do, but both certainly look quite different from the components used to heat a house. The chemical process that our cells utilize to **extract** calories from the food we eat, **calories** to power our activities of living, create heat. Muscle cells, especially, use up a lot of energy and thereby also generate a large percentage of our body's heat. When you go running on a cold day, you do not need a heavy coat to stay warm. When you work hard outside on a hot day, you quickly get very hot. When you feel cold your muscles shiver. That shivering burns calories and thus generates heat. In a real sense your muscles serve as your body's primary furnace.

How about a thermostat? Where would you look for a thermostat inside the human body? What is your best guess?

     ANKLE   APPENDIX   EAR   TONGUE   TOE   BRAIN   LIVER

If you selected the next to the last choice you picked out the correct answer. Not an easy question. The sensing of body temperature and the control for the body's response to being too hot or too cold arise in the hypothalamus, a specific region inside the brain.

FOOD FOR THOUGHT

In the paragraphs above, we used a thermostat controlling a furnace as an example of a control system designed to keep the temperature of a house at a specific value. We picked that example because you have seen thermostats and furnaces, but we would not call that control system very sophisticated. The usual home thermostat turns the furnace on full blast until the room temperature reaches the desired level, then it shuts the furnace completely off. Engineers call that type of controller a "bang-bang controller." "Bang" on, then "bang" off. Guess what happens to the temperature in the room after the furnace shuts off.

Contrast this "bang-bang controller" with the manner in which you might control your bicycle in order to stop precisely where you want to park your bike. You would never pump the peddles at full speed until you reached your destination. Instead you would slow down as you get close and then use your brakes to come to a complete stop at the exact point you desire. If you used the "bang-bang" approach you would expect to fly right by your destination and then have to back up. Exactly that happens each time your furnace gets your house to the desired temperature; it goes a little over and then falls back until the furnace needs to heat up again.

The idea of slowing down or cutting back as you get close to the set point, engineers refer to as proportional control. A proportional controller would represent a more sophisticated or more accurate approach. The design of controllers for all manner of applications has become a specialty in engineering that has a constantly growing set of mathematical tools to guide the design toward ever more accurate and stable controllers. Digital computers make possible controllers that can evoke complex decision-making processes and even change their performance as unexpected situations arise. We call these advanced controllers "learning" or "**adaptive controllers**." Automobiles that drive themselves would represent an example of a very sophisticated adaptive control system capable of adjusting to a wide range of situations.

One can apply the mathematics of control systems to better characterize and understand the processes the human body uses to control its own functions. The specialty of **endocrinology** in medicine focuses almost exclusively on the way the body regulates itself and the conditions in which disease impacts those controls. Physicians do not routinely use mathematics to model those control systems. All specialties of medicine encounter aspects of natural, human control systems that may go astray and thereby create symptoms and abnormal findings.

Man-made controllers have found uses in medical treatment, for example an implanted electronic **pacemaker** used to control the beating of the heart. Numerous other artificial controllers have been designed to solve specific medical problems in drug administration, movement disorders, neural function, and even replacements for lost arms or legs. Most certainly the future will see more and more opportunities to use man-made control systems to replace or augment the control systems the body uses naturally to keep all of our various processes working properly. The human body must have thousands of control systems, many of which we may not currently understand or perhaps even recognize.

The fact that anything we can describe in medicine as having a normal value must have a mechanism for keeping that feature "normal" represents an important concept to keep in your mind.

MEDICAL INVESTIGATION

Medical Investigation 101

Before we started talking about normal values and how they stay normal, you were getting onto an airplane headed to a weekend medical conference. Such **conferences** serve to keep you updated on new information you need to care for your patients. You selected this particular meeting because experts will present new information about how the body controls sleep and on the next day how the body manages aging. Both of these topics come up over and over every day in your office as you deal with your patient's health problems. You feel eager to get to this particular conference.

You do not have one patient complaining of a sleep disturbance; you have dozens. You do not have one patient affected by aging; you do not have any patients not affected by aging. Bright and early Saturday morning you seat yourself right up front ready to soak up any information you can get to improve your care of your patients.

The first speaker has grey hair, which suggests she has studied the topic a long while. The conference moderator finishes his impressive summary of her academic accomplishments, and she begins, "The need for and the purpose of sleep constitute the least clearly understood areas of our research on human sleep." Humans spend about a third of our lives sleeping and we do not know why? Can that really be the case?

Fortunately, the speaker went on to tell her audience a lot of things we do know about sleep. We once thought sleep only served to rest the body, but now we know better. Sleep plays a significant role in learning and long-term memory. Cells inside the brain communicate with each other using electrical impulses, making the brain somewhat akin to a digital computer. While immediate thoughts and actions appear to result from electrical activity inside the brain, long-term memory appears to have chemical aspects that depend upon protein synthesis for the more permanent storage of information (changes in the way the brain cells influence their neighbors). Sleep appears to facilitate the conversion of new information into long-term memory (we learned about backpropogating earlier in investigation 3.13A), but we do not know exactly how. But clearly, when mothers insist their children get plenty of sleep so they can do well in school, science backs up that advice.

The speaker also reviewed a massive amount of information on a center in the brain that times our body's daily activity in sync with the light from the sun and another center that appears to keep tabs on our need to sleep for mind and body rejuvenation. Scientists have studied our brain activity during sleep and defined two main categories of sleep: Rapid eye movement sleep (**REM sleep**) and **non-REM**. The non-REM sleep has three different modes (N1, N2, and N3) and we appear to normally cycle through these stages in steps N1, N2, N3, N2, REM, etc. We dream only during REM sleep. While we think of sleep as a period of resting, during REM sleep some areas of the brain appear to work very hard as indicated by imaging studies that show increases in the blood flowing to those areas, more blood flow than measured when awake.

Sleep seems to occur across the spectrum of animal life. Dolphins, porpoises, and penguins appear able to sleep one half of their brain at a time while the other half remains alert and on guard. Scientists suspect that some birds may have the ability to sleep in flight, but no one has captured direct evidence of this ability. Biologists have studied the sleep patterns of fruit flies and honeybees. Reptiles do not display REM sleep, so they probably do not have nightmares about humans.

But what about those patients who go to their doctor to get help sleeping? The speaker explained that the body has a **biological clock** that readies us to sleep each night. We also have a sense of accumulated physical and mental fatigue that encourages us to sleep. A multitude of factors have the ability to disrupt these natural control systems trying to provide us with sufficient sleep, specifically enough rest, refreshment, and memory assimilation. Disrupted sleep in time becomes chronic sleep deprivation, and that condition can actually sometime require hospitalization to restore a healthy mental functioning. Life events, changes in work schedule, medications, diet changes, or travel across time zones, constitute common causes of sleep disruption.

The speaker noted that sleep scientists have observed that study subjects who get plentiful sleep may not always sleep uninterrupted throughout the night. It would appear that an hour of wakefulness about two-thirds the way through the night occurs commonly enough for them to call that "normal." Those who experience this "wake up" period usually find it not unpleasant and indeed report it seems highly productive as they think about events in their life, often gaining new insights. When patients complain about experiencing sleep disruption, physicians should make sure the complaint does not arise from a norma "wake up" phenomena.

Some medications designed to treat a lack of sleep can themselves disrupt the normal cycle of non-REM and REM sleep, so routine use of these medications can easily become a problem itself. Remember we believe that REM sleep allows the brain to structure long-term memory. Medications the physicians prescribe to treat feelings of depression commonly alter sleep patterns, so physicians need to ask about the sleep experience of patients who are using these medications. The speaker also stressed the importance of a stable sleep schedule and a quiet, dark, comfortable bedroom environment for healthy sleep.

In your role as a physician, take a moment to evaluate the quality of sleep of a patient you know very well: yourself.

How much sleep do you get routinely each night?

Do you have a specific time to go to bed?

Do you dream and remember your dreams?

Do you experience a time during the night of being awake to think?

Do you commonly find yourself feeling very sleepy during the day?

Are there things you want to change to improve the value of your sleep time?

Scientists who study sleep report that individuals who keep a written, daily journal that records every dream they recall upon awaking will find in a few weeks that they will remember multiple dreams in detail each morning. The recall of dreams can often help identify sources of stress in one's life and lead to resolution of those stresses. You might wish to experiment by writing down any dreams you remember each morning.

THE FINAL DAY OF THE CONFERENCE -- FOOD FOR THOUGHT

The last day of the conference introduced a totally new topic. Everyone has an interest in the expectation of the length of his or her life. In the United States we currently expect females to live about 81 years on average and males to live about 76 years. The longest documented human life lasted 122 years. The fact that we can talk about a normal life span for people living in our nation evokes our new rule! If we have a normal value for life span, the human body must have some process that controls it.

On the last day of the conference several speakers talked about life span. In 1993, Dr. Cynthia Kenyon, working at the University of California in San Francisco, discovered that she could modify a **gene** in a particular species of worm she was studying and thus double the lifespan of the worm. The worm did not simply live longer, but actually remained active and vibrant twice as long. Apparently, Dr. Kenyon had successfully slowed the aging process that she previously considered normal for this type of worm.

In 2013, researchers at the National Institutes of Health modified a single gene in a group of mice and extended their average lifespan by about 20%.

In our study of medical science, we have been thinking about medicine and healthcare in terms of diseases that we identify and then treat. But the speakers on this last day of our conference are talking about human aging as a process with a control mechanism we might figure out and modify. Instead of thinking about aging as a normal life process, according to the speakers, medical researchers instead are thinking about aging as a disease we should try to cure.

One of the speakers talked about a drug called **metformin** that physicians use to treat type II diabetes. Studies in animals have demonstrated this drug can slow down aging and studies are underway to test this possibility in humans.

If you were to look up statistics on the average life span of humans in different countries around the world you would find a wide variation. People who live in countries that have limited healthcare and poor living conditions tend to have shorter average life spans. Citizens of wealthier nations currently live longer on average.

Some physicians elect careers in public health. We have not talked about public health as a field of medicine before. Public health professionals primarily focus on the ways that governments or other public institutions can improve the health of their citizens, and the measure of life span can service as a scorecard for public health efforts. The nation of Japan currently appears to lead all others in having the longest average life span among its citizens. Probably many factors contribute to Japan's success, but articles in American medical journals draw attention to a relaxation of mandatory flu shots for school children in

Japan between 1987 and 1994, which resulted in higher death rates across Japan. The Japanese Ministry of Health acted to restore an emphasis on flu shots for both school children and at-risk elderly citizens. School children play a key role in the spread of season flu epidemics and Japan's efforts with regard to this group appear to have played a role in their leading the world in life span statistics as of 2012.

As medical science increases our understanding of what controls aging and how medications might **modulate** those controls, public health may become a very exciting field. The extension of life span within a nation would have major economic effects for governments and on a more individual level would certainly change perspectives on work, personal relationships, family life, and social interactions.

As this weekend conference drew to a close everyone in attendance walked away with a great deal to think about as they traveled home. Take a moment to think about how a dramatic change in life span might impact your life. If you knew at this moment that you would live an active, vibrant life that lasts 120 years, how would your life differ from the life your parents led. If you are going to live to be 120 years old, what might you want to think a lot about?

Investigation 3.14

3.14A: The Final Case
3.14B: Circle of Life

Investigation 3.14A: Final Case

Introduction:

As you study American History you will find the name Dewey pops up again and again. For example, Admiral George Dewey won the Battle of Manila Bay in the Spanish-American War. Melvil Dewey invented the Dewey Decimal System to organize books on library shelves. Thomas Dewey prosecuted infamous gangsters, won election to the office of Governor in the State of New York, but then failed twice to win election to the Presidency of the United States. But focus here for a moment on John Dewey (1859-1982), a college professor, philosopher, psychologist, and educational reformer. John Dewey made his mark in history by challenging teachers not to just teach what they knew, but to provide students with experiences that enable them to teach themselves skills and concepts they will need in their own future. What a challenge!

This book has sought to introduce you to some of the current concepts in medical science, but it has not tried to predict the future of this field of science. To stimulate your interest in medical science as a potential career, we do need to ask about the future. How will medical science change in the coming decades?

Everyone would love to predict the future accurately, but the future has a way of taking turns no one foresees. For readers who indeed are considering healthcare as a potential career choice, gauging the direction of change for the future healthcare has great importance. We do know with great certainty that the future will differ from the present.

Let's try to predict. Let your imagination go wild. If you were to fall ill twenty years in the future, how might healthcare approach your illness? Imagine what that process might involve and jot down some key points? How do you think medical treatment twenty years from now might be different than today?

Did you feel like a science fiction writer? The science fiction stories written years in the past quite often suggested inventions that actually exist today. The comic book character Dick Tracy created many years ago had a ridiculous communicator inside his wristwatch, not too different from the cell phones we find perfectly normal today.

We often foresee the future by looking at **trends** in progress going on today. An example might be found in the treatment of cancer (**oncology**). The term **cancer** refers to diseases in which human cells begin to divide and grow abnormally in numbers and in function. Normal cells have very strong attachments to the cells that surround them, but cancer cells lack that feature, so that they readily spread about the body, a feature we refer to as **metastatic**. Many years ago no treatment existed for cancer. Then mankind learned how to perform surgery and surgeons could remove cancers, but the cancer often **recurred**. Next physicians and medical scientists learned how to attack rapidly growing cancer cells with poisons (**chemotherapy**) and **radiation** (radiation oncology). Since the poisons and radiation they used to attack cancer cells were known also to cause cancer, everyone knew from the beginning those modes of treatment could not possibly prove the optimal therapy in our fight against cancer. We used these treatments because no one had a better solution at the time.

Scientists who studied the biology of human life discovered in the 1950's the molecular structure of our genetic make-up we now all know as DNA. We can find **deoxyribonucleic acid** or DNA in almost every living-cell on earth (the red cells in our blood do not contain DNA). DNA codes direct the manufacturing of **proteins** inside cells (even bacteria). Proteins consist of chains made from 20 **amino acids** and form the complex molecules that make life as we know it possible. The DNA allows living organisms, large and small, to reproduce by making exact copies of their DNA for their offspring. A mistake in copying or an induced defect in a strand of DNA causes both genetic diseases and cancer, and perhaps may also control aging as well.

We know that toxic materials in our environment can create DNA mistakes or defects, as can viral infections, as can radiation to include cosmic rays that travel through space, enter our atmosphere, and pass through our bodies constantly. Mankind has tried to figure out how to eliminate from our environment as many things as possible that can cause cancer, but that effort has provided very limited success. Recently molecular biologists have learned how to modify DNA to allow our body's **immune system** to recognize and kill specific cancer cells without damaging normal cells. They do this by inserting short pieces of DNA into the long DNA strands inside the human cells that fight infections. To do this insertion they use a **modified virus** as the implanting agent. That implanted gene gives the cells of the cancer victim the ability to find and then eliminate the cancer cells that the victim did not previously see as an enemy.

Even more recently scientists working collaboratively in molecular genetics laboratories in the United States and France have discovered a new, simpler method for precisely placing a **genome** into a double stranded DNA molecule. They learned this method by studying the way bacteria acquire immunity to a virus that has infected them. This new method is called CRISPR/Cas9, which stands for Clusters of Regularly Interspaced Short Palindromic Repeats with the Cas9 referring to an associated protein that **cleaves** the DNA at a point programmed by a length of RNA **synthesized** to match the DNA of the target site. Could you make any sense of all those strange words?

While the description of this process sounds complicated a video you can watch on the internet (referenced below) provides a visual image that makes the concept easy to understand. Dr. Jennifer Doudna, who led the development of this remarkable biologic tool, says they have trained high school students in two weeks to successfully **splice** new genes at specified spots inside the DNA of living cells. While gene splicing has been done previously, the CRISPR approach makes the process much easier and more precise. This advance suggests that the ability of medical science to treat diseases with a genetic basis, to include cancer and even infections, will advance now more rapidly than we would previously have predicted. The scientists involved in this work caution the public that making certain that new treatments can do no harm will require years of research. Recently scientists began using CRISPR to modify mosquitos in Brazil in an attempt to reduce their ability to spread diseases such as malaria. Although it will require years to realize the full potential of this technology, knowing of this breakthrough probably helps us view the future of healthcare with more certainty and with great excitement.

Progress in the laboratory of the sort represented by **CRISPR** allows us to also recognize that the list of healthcare providers we have classically considered to include physicians, physician assistants, nurses and nurse practitioners, pharmacists, plus a variety of clinical technicians and technologists, needs alteration. We must include laboratory scientists involved in a **spectrum** of fields that are unlocking the secrets of biology, especially at the molecular level.

Indeed, one can argue that molecular science, not clinical practice, will drive the major advances in medical science in the coming decades.

Take a look at Dr. Jennifer Doudna's presentation on www.ted.com to gain a visual insight into the amazing mechanisms that make this new medical science pathway possible. Direct hands-on clinical care of patients will certainly continue to provide bright minds with highly rewarding careers that combine problem solving based in science with skills in human interaction. But we also want you to appreciate the remarkable discoveries in the laboratory sciences that support the progress in medical practice. These laboratory sciences will likely attract the best and brightest in the years ahead as the frontiers of medical science continue to shift into the domain of molecular biology and chemistry.

Are you surprised to learn that the genetic coding and molecular mechanisms inside a germ are exactly the same as those inside the cells in your body? As you hear Dr. Doudna's presentation jot down other things that surprise you or excite you.

Who would have thought the future of medical science could prove so amazing! Imagine yourself treating patients in what was the future but is now the present. You might find yourself with a whole new arsenal of treatment options that can even cure genetic defects that were untreatable when you were in middle school. Imagine yourself as the treating physician in the following case study.

Case Study

It is quite impressive to look back at the progress humankind has made in the treatment of medical conditions over the past 200 years following many millennia with barely any progress. But looking ahead to the rapid progress that current technology lends to our future medical treatments is even more exiting. The greater the advances we make in technology, the more rapid the advances we make in medical science. Remember the actual definition of technology, "the techniques, methods and processes used in the production of goods or in the accomplishment of scientific objectives." We might view the changes in our Earth itself as moving in the opposite direction. Before man started burning fossil fuels, the atmosphere maintained a consistent composition which comfortably sustained the evolution of life. But the more the planet's population grew, and the more that population burned fossil fuels, the more rapidly changes occurred in our atmosphere. We can only hope that further advances in fuel technology can reverse the rapid changes to our atmosphere that now appear to endanger the very existence of life on our planet.

If you by chance, because of your excitement about this new technology, don't wish to wait until your university molecular biology class to learn more about CRISPR, we recommend you visit the following website:

http://www.yourgenome.org/facts/what-is-crispr-cas9

Investigation 3.14B: Circle of Life

Even as medical research continues to provide new opportunities such as CRISPRS for the treatment of the genetic and infective diseases that plague mankind, the Circle of Life, we do not believe will ever disappear. Death appears inevitable for all living things.

One of the most difficult duties you will have as a physician involves counseling the terminally ill and their families about end of life decisions. When a patient is suffering from extreme difficulty even breathing and having diffuse pain with no reasonable expectation of improvement, the family looks to you for direction on what to do. Some families desire that life be continued as long as possible, while others feel that without some quality of life, life itself may no longer be worthwhile.

Medical Directives are a tool for facilitating the process of determining the degree of medical care desired by the patient himself or herself in those difficult times, when end of life decisions become pertinent. Some assert their desire that no heroic measures, such as surgery or artificial ventilation, be taken to continue their life when little chance exists for restoration of a normal life.

Dr. Hill's family was recently forced to decide the fate of their pet cat, Rudy. Rudy was a happy, active cat for almost thirteen years. Then, suddenly one day, he stopped eating, playing, and socializing; instead he went outside on the deck and stared outward, apparently knowing his life was about to end. We took Rudy to the Vet, who took a history, a blood test, and x-rays. Without doing extensive, expensive testing, she strongly suspected that Rudy had cancer of the liver and would not get better. Sentenced to days of pain and suffering, she advised that they consider **euthanasia** for Rudy.

They took Rudy home, along with pain relieving medicine, so that their children and grand-children could say goodbye. Rudy became a lesson for their grandchildren on the true "Circle of Life"; everyone cried and wished Rudy a pleasant journey to Kitty Heaven.

The next day they returned to the veterinary clinic, where they experienced a most compassionate and peaceful end to Rudy's life. As Rudy labored to breathe, the Vet gave Rudy a sedative that allowed him to fall asleep as they stroked his fur and spoke peacefully to him. After he was totally unconscious, the Vet gave the final injection, and within a minute confirmed that Rudy was no longer of this life.

We hope that one-day, most, if not all humans can end their lives in peaceful slumber, such as Rudy did. Unfortunately, we cannot always choose the time and place where our lives end; even having the ability to alter genes does not protect us from tragedies. Therefore, we should strive to live each day as though it could be our last. Do something you are proud of each day! Offer help to someone in need; treat others with respect. Make your world a kinder, gentler world. Practice the art of compassion; you will find it very useful in your life whether or not you choose a career in medicine.

Investigation 3.15: Looking Deeper

Investigation 3.15: Looking Deeper

Introduction:

The basic structure of medical investigation this book has introduced to you involves putting the information surrounding a patient's complaint into a specific format called the **History and Physical**. We then add information from other tests and evaluations in order to separate out the correct diagnosis from a list we have called the **Differential Diagnosis**, all the possible causes for the symptoms the patient exhibits. Do doctors actually go through that process all day long with every patient they see? You probably have realized by now based on your own experiences, they do not.

Physicians see patients day after day who have very similar problems. Since physicians specialize in particular areas of the body, the spectrum of problems that come to them has shrunk through the efforts of emergency room or general practice physicians who tend to make referrals to more specialized physicians. Over time physicians tend to use their **experience** to jump quickly to the right diagnosis without formally working through a differential diagnosis list.

It is important to remember the practice of medicine is as much 'art' as it is science. Physicians must merge their scientific knowledge of anatomy, physiology, and pathology with all of the information their examinations and testing have accumulated about this specific patient's medical problem. Doctors find themselves asking why again and again in the course of solving each medical investigation. Why does the patient show these particular symptoms? What could cause this abnormal test result? Getting to the correct answer often requires deep, probing thought; yet we have also seen that physicians do not always reach the correct diagnosis.

We created this book to introduce you to the world of healthcare and perhaps to invite you to consider such a career for yourself. Also, we want you to benefit from a better understanding of how people go about solving real-life problems.

You can use the structure of the medical history and physical and the differential diagnosis as a template for thinking about problems in other areas of your life. People in many fields make decisions by writing down what they know about a problem in a formal way and then writing down possible actions or explanations that they can then test in order to make the best decision.

Seeing that the medical decision process we outlined above fails from time to time, we might also profit by expecting that our initial decisions in life can go wrong and need re-evaluation. This sort of real world experience can prove valuable no matter what path we choose for our life.

Tom Brokaw's name may not sound familiar to you, but probably would to your parents. Brokaw visited millions of American homes every evening to deliver the news of the day on network television. Doing that made him almost a member of the family in many homes. Brokaw retired from television to a ranch in Montana. He stayed active on the ranch with occasional television appearances until he began to experience persistent back pain. As a famous American he had access to great doctors and saw a couple renowned orthopedic surgeons who set about to treat his back pain. Brokaw wrote about this in a book he titled, <u>A Lucky Life, Interrupted</u>. The renowned physicians did not consider all the possible causes of back pain before jumping to a diagnosis and treatment plan, and in fact Brokaw's primary care physician ultimately stepping in to get him the right diagnosis and the right treatment by looking deeper. Brokaw needed a totally different set of physicians to solve his real problem.

You have read in this book about a patient who has chest pain. Working from the initial symptoms a number of possible causes could explain the patient's pain, but then the next day that patient developed a rash along one of his ribs that made the diagnosis of shingles quite obvious. Having made the diagnosis, we treated him for shingles. But did we ask, why did he have shingles? We did not stop to ask ourselves what caused his immune system to suddenly allow the chickenpox virus to again attack his body. We failed to "think deeper."

Medical Investigation 101

Some have called **Sakichi Toyoda** (1867 – 1930) the "King of Japanese inventors." He founded the Japanese company Toyota, still a company well known as a powerhouse of innovation today in motor vehicles. We credit Sakichi Toyoda with the creation of a trick for thinking deeper called "**5 Whys**." He believed in order to find creative solutions to problems one must dig down to the root of the problem, and not be content with the superficial cause of an issue. In the 5 Whys method one asks why, and then subjects the answer to that question to another level of asking why. You try to do this process five times. We do not know exactly why he picked the number five, because frequently one cannot readily dig that deeply. Instead focus your attention on asking why repeatedly as many times as you can to force yourself to think deeper and deeper into a problem you face.

Let's try an example:

1. Why is the sky blue? Sunlight is white so when we look at the sky something must have removed the red end of the color spectrum leaving the blue light behind.

2. Why would the blue light separate out? At sunset sometimes the sun looks red, so in that case the blue light has been subtracted along the direct path from my eye to the sun.

3. Why would the blue light not stay with the red? I looked that up and it seems dust in the atmosphere scatters out the lower frequency light more easily than the higher frequencies.

4. Why would dust act this way on light? We have asked why only four times and now find ourselves asking a question appropriate for a college physics class.

Maybe Sakichi Toyoda really had a great idea. We would probably have been better physicians if we asked ourselves why our patient with shingles got shingles. The answer to that question may have opened doors into early treatment of problems that had not yet created symptoms for our patient.

We are going to leave you to try out the "**5-Whys**." The question can be anything you want to think about from, "Why does my brother yell at me?" to "Why do I need a belt to hold up my pants?" You pick the question and see what happens as you ask why of each answer, trying to repeat this process five times, taking you deeper and deeper into the question.

A 7th grade student came up with the following example when asked to think deeper using the 5-Whys:

Question #1: Why do I have to go to school?

Answer: To get an education

Question #2: Why do I need an education?

Answer: So I can get a good job

Question #3: Why do I need a good job?

Answer: So I can make good money

Question #4: Why do I need to make good money?

Answer: So I can pay my bills

Question #5: Why do I need to pay my bills?

Answer: So I can raise a family and be happy

Not only did that exercise force him to think about why he was at school, it caused him to relate the quality of his future life to his effort and achievement in school today. Getting kids to think into their future is not always easy in this "think about the moment" world in which we live.

Medical Investigation 101

Now you try.

Directions: Here is your opportunity to practice thinking deeper about a question on *your* mind. Your challenge is to: 1. Think of a 'why' question, then 2. Answer that question. 3. Ask 'why' that answer is true. You will then pose a 'why' question about your answer to question #2. At this point you have already reached level three depth thinking. Your ultimate challenge is to see if you can get to level five; but don't be too disappointed if you get stuck somewhere in the middle of this process. Refer back to our example if you need a refresher on the mechanics of deeper thinking. Notice that we only got a level 4 in our example before we needed outside help.

Deeper thinking is not easy and learning to use it requires practice. But think for a moment about the benefits you will gain by utilizing deeper thinking in the important choices you consider and decisions you make going forward. Set up your paper to think deeper like the following example.

Deeper Thinking Activity

Why Question #1: _____
Answer: _____

Why Question #2: _____
Answer: _____

Why Question #3: _____
Answer: _____

Why Question #4: _____
Answer: _____

Why Question #5: _____
Answer: _____

Sakichi Toyoda left us a great tool for deep thinking.

Post-Script

Congratulations! You have successfully completed a journey into the world of the medical practitioner. You now have a better understanding of the thought process required to solve the medical investigations so important and meaningful to your patients' well-being. This same process of asking "why" and looking deeper can work in your daily life as a student and well beyond as you strive to make good life decisions.

You also appreciate now that, regardless of your future occupation, solving significant problems of all types often requires collaboration and teamwork. Complex issues benefit from the input of people with a diversity of training, experience, and insight. In almost any career you will work with others to find the successful solutions to the challenges you face. Individuals you trust can prove essential for even personal problems you may face in the years ahead. Many successful people actually create their own personal "Board of Directors" to call on for advice when they make important decisions. We wish you a successful journey as you solve the challenges and investigations in your life. No life completely avoids stress and difficulty, but we hope some of the lessons you have learned in this introduction to medical investigation make you better able to make sound decisions. Thanks for allowing us into your life.

About the Authors:

In his youth **Dr. Russ Hill** imagined himself playing professional baseball, encouraged by a successful high school baseball career. But higher levels of competition failed to ratify that expectation, so he had to pursue his backup plan. In college he trained for teaching, but upon graduation no jobs were open. Instead he found an opportunity in pharmaceutical sales. While doing that work he met a Podiatrist who was an alumnus of Dr. Hill's own high school. The doctor challenged him to further his science education and then apply to Podiatry school. He did and at the end of a career in health care he retired, still feeling the need for challenges in his life.

In pursuit of another challenge, Dr. Hill followed his daughter into the teaching profession, a profession he originally had pursued over twenty years earlier. Over the past decade and a half he has challenged his students to bump up their own aspirations, just as the Podiatrist had done for him. He still teaches middle school Science and STEM.

The current trend in education has put a focus on career readiness, and yet we have not seen a textbook that introduces students to medically-oriented careers. This one tries to do just that by providing insights into how doctors analyze problems and conduct medical investigations. Whether students end up with a medically oriented career or not, the analytical skills required of physicians have applications in almost all careers we expect to see opening up in the future. Besides, It never hurts to have some basic medical knowledge tucked away when collaborating with a physician to maintain your own good health.

Dr. Richard Griffith never imagined a career in medicine when he was your age. Instead electronics fascinated him at a time when America was very excited about going into outer space. He took math and physics in a small town high school from a former mining engineer who encouraged him to ask why, and challenge the simple answers to questions. In college he studied physics, but eventually recognized that his passion lay in solving everyday problems and not so much finding new sub-atomic particles. He went to graduate school in electrical engineering and got interested in medical applications for engineering tools. He got career guidance from an older engineer who had attended medical school and eventually became a researcher at the National Institutes of Health. Based on his advice, Griffith completed a doctorate in electrical engineering and then applied to medical school, frankly not expecting to get accepted since biology and chemistry were not a significant part of his prior studies. To his surprise they let him in and he managed to transition into this very different mode of thinking and learning.

His electrical engineering background got him involved in research in neurosurgery even before he finished medical school, but he decided that he needed a clinical specialty for a successful career, so he selected a residency in anesthesiology. That specialty seemed to best suit his array of interests. He since has done private practice, worked as a medical director in a major medical device company, and finally finished his career in academic medicine teaching medical students and resident physicians. Now retired in Vermont, he has been working to involve industrial designers more fully in the cause of Patient Safety, because mistakes in health care have become an alarmingly common occurrence despite the best intentions of health care professionals. It appears that industrial designers have some unique skills that may prove especially valuable in the future of safer medical care.

Russ Hill and Richard Griffith are First Cousins who grew up on opposite sides of this country, Griffith in Virginia and Hill in California. Griffith's Mother was the Sister of Hill's Father. Griffith was thirteen and Hill was eleven when they first met. Griffith's family had driven west for his Father to attend a summer workshop in economics and to visit their distant Hill relatives. They made that 6,000 miles round trip in the middle of summer with no radio or air conditioner in their car. Times were tough back then. The two cousins did not see one other in person again until seventeen years later when Hill's family visited the Griffith family in Virginia. In the ensuing years they have communicated by email as their friendship grew. They have gotten together a few times in New York, Montana, and Vermont, where Griffith now lives. In spite of the geographical barrier, they successfully collaborated by many e-mails for over a year in order to write this book.

Raella Hill married Russ more than 45 years ago, first meeting him in high school. She worked in hospitals before taking several years off to raise her two children. She then studied art and immersed herself in ceramics, photography, painting, and printmaking. Her final career job was as office manager for architectural photographers. Her interests now include her four grandchildren, printmaking, and yoga.

Medical Investigation 101

Medical Investigation 101 can be read independently or utilized in conjunction with the workbook for best results. *Medical Investigation 101 Workbook* was designed for those interested in an interactive experience that reinforces the information and concepts discussed in the book. *Medical Investigation 101 Teacher's Edition* provides the answers to the questions, crossword puzzles, and activities from the workbook.

ISBN Number	Book
9781548510466	*Medical Investigation 101 Workbook*: Interactive Assignments Aligned with Medical Investigation 101
9781974284863	*Medical Investigation 101 Workbook*: **Teacher's Edition**

Notes about things I want to remember or understand better.

Made in the USA
Monee, IL
01 September 2021